Overview of:

HEALTHCARE
COMPLIANCE

Sarah Godwin Brinson   Lesley Clack
Larecia Money Gill   Laura Kim Gosa

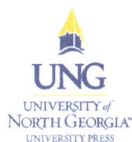

UNG

UNIVERSITY *of*
NORTH GEORGIA™
UNIVERSITY PRESS

Blue Ridge | Cumming | Dahlonega | Gainesville | Oconee

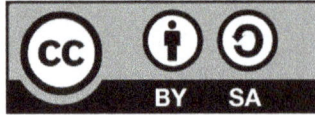

ISBN: 978-1-940771-85-4

Produced by:
University System of Georgia

Published by:
University of North Georgia Press
Dahlonega, Georgia

Cover Design: Alexa Hernandez-Lopez
Layout Design: Corey Parson

For more information, please visit http://ung.edu/university-press
Or email ungpress@ung.edu

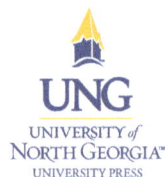

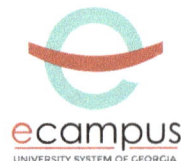

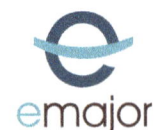

TABLE OF CONTENTS

HEALTH INSURANCE & REIMBURSEMENT 30

QUALITY IMPROVEMENT 55

STRATEGIC PLANNING   68

MANAGING HEALTHCARE PROFESSIONALS & STRATEGIC
MANAGEMENT OF HUMAN RESOURCES   80

HEALTHCARE TECHNOLOGY 92

SPECIAL TOPICS AND EMERGING ISSUES IN HEALTHCARE MANAGEMENT 115

1

Introduction to Healthcare Compliance

1.1 LEARNING OBJECTIVES

1. Describe how the U.S. has become a major player in global health and what role healthcare compliance plays in the healthcare industry.

2. Explain how a healthcare compliance program works.

3. Discuss why compliance programs are important to healthcare organizations.

4. Discuss the benefits of initiating a healthcare compliance program.

1.2 INTRODUCTION

The United States has been at the forefront of globalized health care for many years by influencing international healthcare policy and establishing international healthcare agencies to address global health threats such as HIV/AIDS, tuberculosis, and malaria. It has also been a leader in medical innovation and technology over the past two decades, a time of many changes in the world of healthcare. Due to these changes, the rules, regulations, and legislation are also constantly changing, making healthcare compliance a challenge. This chapter will discuss the rise of U.S. healthcare on the global stage, define healthcare compliance, and discuss penalties for noncompliance.

1.3 KEY TERMS

- Centers for Medicare and Medicaid Services (CMS)
- Chief Executive Officer (CEO)
- Compliance Officer
- Healthcare compliance
- Office of Inspector General (OIG)
- Third-Party Payer

1.4 THE HISTORY OF HEALTHCARE IN THE UNITED STATES

With the compliance minded industry and standards of today's healthcare in mind, it is difficult to imagine a time when the United States was not the highly regulated powerhouse of medical technology and innovation that it is now. However, prior to the 18th century, health care in the U.S. was practiced informally with little training required. By the late 1700s, medical schools began appearing in the U.S. which provided formalized training for physicians.

In the late 1700s, the industrial revolution also began in the U.S. and lasted over a century. With the industrial revolution came an increase of jobs in steel mills and with the railroad. Coincidentally, job-related injuries increased due to the nature of this work. Increase in injuries further occurred due to the U.S.'s involvement in numerous wars. These events compelled healthcare practitioners to develop innovative medical treatments—and thus launched the U.S.'s global dominance in healthcare technology and innovation.

During the 19th and 20th centuries, American scientists and physicians developed medical breakthroughs ranging from immunizations and antibiotics to surgical and cardiovascular treatments. These treatments soon spread internationally and became the standard of care worldwide. As medical advances continued, the U.S. realized their impact on a global scale and the importance of ensuring these treatments were available to all global citizens. This realization inspired the U.S. to invest in global health initiatives such as HIV/AIDS relief and immunization programs. Many view foreign aid simply as support for the international community; however, the U.S. recognizes this aid assists more than the recipient country. Foreign aid prevents pandemic outbreaks of infectious diseases and promotes increased productivity and economic growth internationally (National Academy of Sciences, 2017). By improving the health and financial stability of global citizens, the U.S. protects American citizens located both abroad and at home.

The U.S. attracts the world's smartest and most talented scientist and researchers by offering financial incentives provided by our capitalist system. Capitalism allows for efficient allocation of resources and production and a creative and economic freedom not available in all countries; it also drives business and profits within the U.S. (Pettinger, 2019). Because of these advantages, the U.S. leads the world in medical technology and treatments, as shown through their state-of-the-art medical facilities, advanced treatment protocols, and access to technology and innovation in U.S. facilities (Thorpe, 2011).

1.5 HEALTHCARE COMPLIANCE

Over the last two decades, the healthcare industry has experienced stable growth for several reasons, including population growth, population aging, disease prevalence, medical advancements, and utilization of services (Probasco, 2019). Due to advances in medical treatment, the average lifespan of most people has been extended. Consequently, healthcare providers are caring for patients who are older with more comorbidities than in years past. Healthcare providers are also seeing these patients in diverse care settings, including health clinics, physician's offices, hospitals, and domestic spaces. In order to receive reimbursement, health care providers must adhere to the laws, policies, and procedures that are in place to regulate these care settings. However, many agencies regulate these care practices, including federal and state legislatures and administrative agencies, such as the Internal Revenue Service (IRS), the Department of Health and Human Services (HHS), and the Centers for Medicare and Medicaid Services (CMS) (Safian, 2009). These agencies guide and inform healthcare providers of their responsibilities in providing patient care, including reimbursement practices.

Due to the sheer number of laws, policies, and regulatory agencies in place to keep up with the healthcare industry's growth, it is difficult to understand, much less remain compliant with, the standards of practice. In order to ensure compliance with these regulations, healthcare facilities have developed compliance programs. These programs interpret laws and regulations and translate them into language that healthcare providers can understand. After this process has occurred, members of the compliance team (usually referred to as compliance officers) then educate staff—including health care professionals—on how these laws and regulations impact their health care practice. A compliance program also develops policies regarding how violations are reported and determines what sanctions will be enforced for noncompliance. Therefore, compliance programs have three distinct roles: prevention, detection, and correction (Hartunian, Wolff, & Seigel, 2018). According to the Office of Inspector General (2011), seven key elements of a compliance program fit under each of the roles:

1.5.1 Role 1, Prevention:

1. *Written policies/procedures*: all policies and procedures should be located in a document that is readily accessible to all employees of the organization. Along with the policies and procedures, there should be information included in this document that details the implementation and operation of the compliance program.

2. *Compliance professionals*: the organization should designate a compliance officer to oversee the organization's compliance efforts. This individual needs to have enough autonomy and authority to conduct the position's duties without interference. This position should report directly to the Chief Executive Officer (CEO) and/or the Board of Directors. A compliance committee should also be in place and meet at least twice per year to review any grievances filed and quality reports (which are required as part of the internal auditing process).

3. *Effective training*: once policies and procedures are in place, the compliance officer should implement a training program with all

employees that covers general compliance issues; fraud, waste, and abuse; the Anti-Kickback Statute (AKS); the False Claims Act; and the issue of inappropriate gifts/relationships with referral sources (Hartunian, Wolff, & Seigel, 2018). The training should be documented and offered upon hiring and annually thereafter.

4. ***Effective communication***: in addition to training, employees should be informed of confidential, anonymous ways they can report compliance concerns. This may be achieved by offering a hotline or an email address that should be shared with all employees using multiple methods (i.e., email, printed flyer, etc.).

1.5.2 Role 2, Detection:

5. ***Internal monitoring***: in addition to regularly monitoring the compliance hotline, the compliance officer should also perform an annual risk assessment. This assessment includes regular meetings with staff to identify risks, compliance challenges, and areas of noncompliance. A written report should be developed and presented to senior leadership, along with strategies to address these issues and avoid future violations.

1.5.3 Role 3, Corrective Action:

6. ***Enforcement of standards:*** disciplinary approaches that are consistently applied to all employees should be outlined in the compliance program. Anyone found to violate the compliance standards by participating in unlawful or unethical actions should be terminated.

7. ***Prompt response:*** investigations of reported noncompliance must be conducted quickly to avoid a False Claim Act (FCA) case. Organizations have sixty days from the time a violation is reported to respond in cases of overpayment.

Real-Life Example

In 2018, the U.S. Department of Justice (US DOJ) prosecuted the largest healthcare fraud case in history. The nationwide case involved 58 districts and 601 defendants (including 165 doctors, nurses, and other professionals) who filed approximately $2 billion in false claims and 30 state Medicaid Fraud Control Units (MFCUs). Of those charged, 76 physicians were indicted for prescribing and distributing opioids and other narcotics, and 2,700 individuals were excluded from participating in Medicare, Medicaid, and all other federal healthcare programs (US DOJ, 2018). The government has indicated its level of support for preventing Medicare and Medicaid fraud, waste, and abuse by including $751 million in funding for monitoring and investigating such cases for fiscal year 2018 (Hartunian, Wolff, & Seigel, 2017).

Source: Manatt
Attribution: (Hartunian, Wolff, & Seigel, 2017)
License: Fair Use

1.6 BENEFITS OF COMPLIANCE PROGRAMS

Health care is dynamic and constantly changing, with medical advancements occurring daily. Along with these advancements come updated rules, regulations, and laws. It is impossible for healthcare facilities to remain knowledgeable of these changes and compliant with the multitudes of regulatory agencies that oversee the implementation and compliance of these changes. Therefore, instituting a compliance program that will monitor for these changes and implement any needed program revisions to ensure compliance is a major benefit. In addition to monitoring for changes, compliance officers interpret the rules, regulations, and laws, and provide written guidelines that are easily understood. They then educate all staff members on the guidelines, monitor for adherence, and provide corrective measures before regulatory agencies are alerted and/or issue sanctions. Compliance programs also offer staff an internal means for reporting violations.

Outcomes of effective compliance programs include increased staff knowledge and adherence to regulations, improved safety and service to patients, and reduced liability resulting in increased revenue (Safian, 2009). Staff cannot adhere to rules and regulations of which they are unaware. However, ignorance of the regulation is not a defense, as most laws are written using the phrase "knows or *should know*." Therefore, it is essential that healthcare organizations ensure that staff are properly educated on their responsibilities; often, this task is a requirement of the laws themselves. However, this information must be explained in an easily understood manner so as to avoid any possible confusion that may lead to inadvertent violations.

Health care compliance thus leads to improved patient safety and service due to strict adherence to established policies and procedures. These policies and procedures cover services ranging from medical coding to patient care documentation. Each of these services contributes to positive patient outcomes by ensuring the patient's diagnosis is documented accurately and the patient receives the appropriate medical care related to the diagnosis. By complying with the policies and procedures, the risk of committing a medical error is reduced and the likelihood of negative patient outcomes decreased.

Each year, approximately 400,000 patients who are hospitalized experience harm from *preventable* medical errors (James, 2013). These errors result in the deaths of over 100,000 people annually and cost approximately $20 billion per year in such direct costs as litigation and patient treatments due to medical errors and such indirect costs as decreased productivity and staff absenteeism related to event investigations and court appearances (Blair, 2012; Ditmer, 2010; Neilsen & Einarsen, 2012). An additional consequence of noncompliance is lost revenue due to facility and/or physician exclusion from participation with Medicare, Medicaid, or other third-party payers. Decreasing medical errors lessens the chances of developing negative patient outcomes, which results in fewer lawsuits and a reduced loss of revenue. One solution to address this potential problem is to implement and uphold a culture of safety that adheres to prescribed standards of care (Rodziewicz & Hipskind, 2019). Healthcare compliance programs are one way to ensure your organization is practicing within the confines of the law and maintaining this culture of safety. Compliance programs also convey the organization's intent to adhere to policies, procedures, and laws. The very existence of a compliance program within an organization may result in lower penalties and fines if an organization is found guilty of violating federal laws.

1.7 COMPLIANCE DOCUMENTATION

In health care, the basic rule of "if it is not documented then you did not do it" is the golden rule regarding compliance. It doesn't matter if your facility is 100% compliant with regulations; if it isn't documented then you are considered noncompliant. The benefits of documentation are evident: documentation lends support for compliance! However, other benefits may not be as evident; for instance, documentation provides information to assist with decision making for patient care and provides a means for communication between providers to ensure continuity of patient care and increased patient safety (Safian, 2009). Documentation can also lead to public safety measures by identifying trends in illnesses and outcomes of health promotion programs. This data can also be used when conducting research to assist in determining the most effective treatment modalities and to develop updated care protocols. Based on data (documentation) collected, organizations can determine how to distribute equipment, staff, finances (i.e., budget), and other resources to ensure they are allocated appropriately and equitably based on the department's needs (Sabian, 2009). Documentation can also be reviewed to identify areas of potential risks and guide quality improvement measures. One additional benefit of documentation is accurately reflecting patients' diagnoses and treatments rendered for billing purposes. If patient visits are not documented accurately, then they will not be coded properly, which will affect reimbursement for the visit. More importantly, if the payer reimbursed the physician and/or organization for incorrect treatments and/or diagnoses, the offending agent can be charged with making false claims and fined (including repaying any monies received), charged with criminal acts, risk incarceration, and/or lose the ability to participate in treating Medicare/Medicaid patients.

False Claim Act

Liability

The statute begins, in § 3729(a), by explaining the conduct that creates FCA liability. In very general terms, §§ 3729(a)(1)(A) and (B) set forth FCA liability for any person who knowingly submits a false claim to the government or causes another to submit a false claim to the government or knowingly makes a false record or statement to get a false claim paid by the government. Section 3729(a)(1)(G) is known as the reverse false claims section; it provides liability where one acts improperly—not to get money from the government but to avoid having to pay money to the government. Section 3729(a)(1)(C) creates liability for those who conspire to violate the FCA. Sections 3729(a)(1)(D), (E), and (F) are rarely invoked. Damages and penalties: After listing the seven types of conduct that result in FCA liability, the statute provides that one who is liable must pay a civil penalty of between $5,000 and $10,000 for each false claim (those amounts are adjusted from time to time; the current amounts are $5,500 to $11,000) and treble the amount of the government's damages. If a person who has violated the FCA reports the incident to the government under certain conditions, the FCA provides that the person shall be liable for not less than double the damages.
The knowledge requirement: A person does not violate the False Claims Act by submitting a false claim to the government unwittingly; to violate the FCA a person must have submitted, or caused the submission of, the false claim (or made a false statement or record) with knowledge of the falsity. In § 3729(b)(1), knowledge of false information is defined as being (1) actual knowledge, (2) deliberate ignorance of the truth or intentionally falsifying information, or (3) reckless disregard of the truth or falsifying information.

(Department of Justice, 2011)

Source: The United States Department of Justice
Attribution: The United States Department of Justice
License: Public Domain

All individuals who document in a patient's record are responsible for providing complete, accurate records that are easily accessible to others involved in the patient's care (Safian, 2009). The importance of this procedure cannot be understated: the inclusion and/or exclusion of vital information may impact third-party payers' decisions to reimburse providers and/or organizations for services. For example, the Centers for Medicare and Medicaid Services (CMS) published a list of "never events" for which they will not pay for care associated with such events. Incidents such as operating on the wrong body part, leaving a foreign body in a patient after surgery, severe pressure ulcers, and mismatched blood transfusions are examples of "never events." These events are costly to the healthcare facility, which must cover all costs associated with each occurrence. For example, catheter associated urinary tract infections (CAUTIs) are considered to be hospital acquired infections and cost up to $29,743 per occurrence to treat (Agency for Healthcare Research and Quality, 2017).

Case Example

Mrs. Jones, a 72-year-old female, is admitted to the hospital with a diabetic ketoacidosis diagnosis. Upon admission to the ICU, the admitting nurse fails to document a pressure ulcer that was located in Mrs. Jones' lower back. The next day, the nurse assigned to care for Mrs. Jones discovers the pressure ulcer and documents it in her assessment. Because the pressure ulcer was not properly identified and documented upon admission, CMS considers this condition as a hospital acquired state and, therefore, refuses to pay the charges associated with care rendered for this problem.

Source: Original Work
Attribution: Larecia Gill
License: CC BY-SA 4.0

Documentation must also be completed in a timely manner. With the national mandate for the use of electronic health records (EHR) by all physicians and organizations who treat patients covered by governmental insurance, documentation is recorded in real time, thus entries are time stamped (Atherton, 2011). Therefore, providers can no longer document when it is convenient for them but must record their assessments and treatment plans in the immediate period following the patient encounter. Along with these essential elements, providers must also confirm the entry was created by them by providing their signature (either electronically or manually) (Safrian, 2009).

Another essential component of documentation is legibility. This issue has been greatly improved with the implementation of EHR. However, it is still important for providers to be knowledgeable on approved abbreviations for use in documentation. The Joint Commission (2019) developed a list of unapproved abbreviations that should never be used when documenting. They also provide a list of abbreviations, acronyms, and symbols that should be used with extreme caution due to the high risk of confusion and/or misinterpretation. Each organization determines which abbreviations to include on their "Do Not Use" list. Therefore, healthcare professionals are responsible for knowing these institutional policies.

5

Do Not Use	Potential Problem	Use Instead
U (unit)	Mistaken for "0" (zero), the number "4" (four) or "cc"	Write "unit"
IU (International Unit)	Mistaken for IV (intravenous) or the number 10 (ten)	Write "International Unit"
Q.D., QD, q.d., qd(daily)	Mistaken for each other	Write "daily"
Q.O.D., QOD, q.o.d, qod (every other day)	Period after the Q mistaken for "I" and the "O" mistaken for "I"	Write "every other day
Trailing zero (X.0 mg)* Lack of leading zero (.X mg)	Decimal point is missed	Write X mg Write 0.X mg
MS	Can mean morphine sulfate or magnesium sulfate	Write "morphine sulfate" Write "magnesium sulfate"
MSO4 and MgSO4	Confused for one another	Write "morphine sulfate" Write "magnesium sulfate"
*Exception: A "trailing zero" may be used only where required to demonstrate the level of precision of the value being reported, such as for laboratory results, imaging studies that report size of lesions, or catheter/tube sizes. It may not be used in medication orders or other medication-related documentation.		

Table 1.1: The Joint Commission Official "Do Not Use" List (2019)

Source: The Joint Commission
Attribution: The Joint Commission
License: © The Joint Commission, 2021. Reprinted with permission.

Do Not Use	Potential Problem	Use Instead
> (greater than) < (less than)	Misinterpreted as the number "7" (seven) or the letter "L" Confused for one another	Write "greater than" Write "less than"
Abbreviations for drug names	Misinterpreted due to similar abbreviations for multiple drugs	Write drug names in full

Apothecary units	Unfamiliar to many practitioners Confused with metric units	Use metric units
@	Mistaken for the number "2" (two)	Write "at"
cc	Mistaken for U (units) when poorly written	Write "mL" or "ml" or "milliliters" ("mL" is preferred)
µg	Mistaken for mg (milligrams) resulting in one thousand-fold overdose	Write "mcg" or "micrograms"

Table 1.2: Additional Abbreviations, Acronyms and Symbols (For possible future inclusion in the Official "Do Not Use" List)

Source: The Joint Commission

Attribution: The Joint Commission

License: © The Joint Commission, 2021. Reprinted with permission.

Regardless of the setting where a patient encounter occurs, certain details must be included to meet compliance regulations, such as the following:

- Date of patient encounter
- Identification of patient: including patient's full name, address, phone number, date of birth, and emergency contact information
- Internal patient identifier (i.e., medical record number, patient number)
- Identification of treating provider
- Reason(s) for encounter (i.e., diagnosis, chief complaint)
- Details of encounter:
  - ◇ Subjective Data (based on personal opinion, interpretation, point of view):
    - Discussions
    - Communications
    - History of present illness (HPI)
    - Past medical history (PMH)
    - Family and social history
    - Allergies
    - Medications
    - Previous surgeries

◇ Objective Data (fact-based, measurable and observable):

- Findings of physical examination

- Labs or procedures (with results)

- Healthcare provider's interpretation/diagnoses, including any prescriptions provided and recommendations for follow-up

• Healthcare provider's signature

(Department of Justice, 2011)

ESSENTIAL COMPONENTS OF DOCUMENTATION

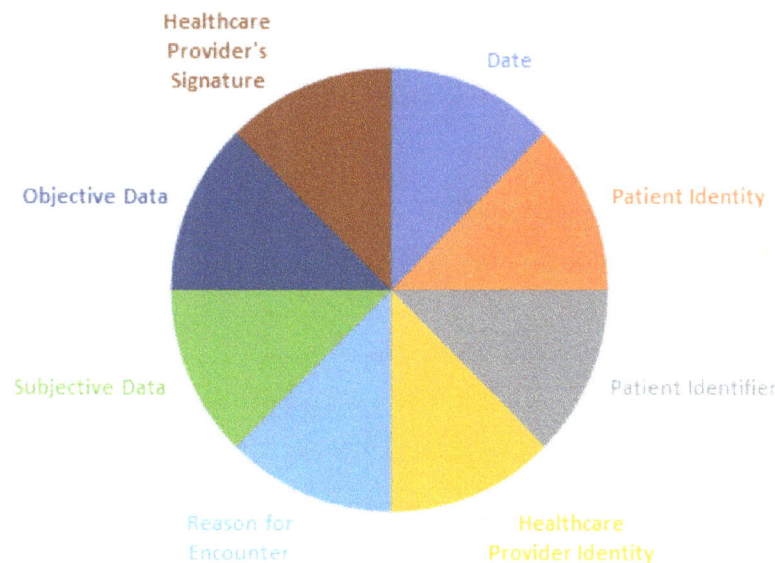

Figure 1.1: Essential Components of Documentation

Source: Original Work
Attribution: Larecia Gill
License: CC BY-SA 4.0

Laws and accrediting bodies may require elements in addition to the ones stated above to meet compliance regulations. For example, the False Claim Act requires that documentation demonstrates medical necessity for a prescribed treatment, service, or medical equipment (Department of Justice, 2011). Certificates of Medical Necessity (CMN) must be completed by the prescribing healthcare provider before third-party payers will pay for the service/equipment. An example of a CMN appears on the following pages.

DEPARTMENT OF HEALTH AND HUMAN SERVICES
CENTERS FOR MEDICARE & MEDICAID SERVICES

Form Approved
OMB No. OMB 0938-0679

CERTIFICATE OF MEDICAL NECESSITY   DME 03.03

CMS-10269: POSITIVE AIRWAY PRESSURE (PAP) DEVICES FOR OBSTRUCTIVE SLEEP APNEA

SECTION A: Certification Type/Date: INITIAL____/___/____RECERTIFICATION____/___/___

PATIENT NAME, ADDRESS, TELEPHONE and HICN	SUPPLIER NAME, ADDRESS, TELEPHONE and NSC or NPI #
(_____) _____ HICN _____	(_____) _____ NSC or NPI # _____

PLACE OF SERVICE _____	HCPCS CODE	PT DOB____/___/___ ; Sex____(M/F) ; HT_____(in.) ; WT_____(lbs.)
NAME and ADDRESS of FACILITY if applicable (See Reverse)		PHYSICIAN NAME, ADDRESS (Printed or Typed)
		PHYSICIAN'S NSC or NPI #: _____
		PHYSICIAN'S TELEPHONE #: (_____) _____

SECTION B: Information in this section may not be completed by the supplier of the items/supplies.

EST. LENGTH OF NEED (# OF MONTHS):_____ 1–99 (99=LIFETIME) DIAGNOSIS CODES (ICD-9): _____ _____ _____ _____

ANSWERS	ANSWER QUESTIONS 1–7 FOR INITIAL EVALUATION
	ANSWER QUESTIONS 8–10 FOR FOLLOW-UP EVALUATION (RECERTIFICATION)
	(Check Y for Yes, N for No, D for Does Not Apply)
☐Y ☐N	1. Is the device being ordered for the treatment of obstructive sleep apnea (ICD-9 diagnosis code 327.23)? If YES, continue to Questions 2–5; If NO, Proceed to Section D
___/___/___	2. Enter date of initial face-to-face evaluation
___/___/___	3. Enter date of sleep test (If test spans multiple days, enter date of first day of test)
☐Y ☐N	4. Was the patient's sleep test conducted in a facility-based lab?
_____	5. What is the patient's Apnea-Hypopnea Index (AHI) or Respiratory Disturbance Index (RDI)?
☐Y ☐N	6. Does the patient have documented evidence of at least one of the following? Excessive daytime sleepiness, impaired cognition, mood disorders, insomnia, hypertension, ischemic heart disease or history of stroke.
☐Y ☐N ☐D	7. If a bilevel device is ordered, has a CPAP device been tried and found ineffective?
___/___/___	8. Enter date of follow-up face-to-face evaluation.
☐Y ☐N	9. Is there a report documenting that the patient used PAP ≥ 4 hours per night on at least 70% of nights in a 30 consecutive day period?
☐Y ☐N	10. Did the patient demonstrate improvement in symptoms of obstructive sleep apnea with the use of PAP?

NAME OF PERSON ANSWERING SECTION B QUESTIONS, IF OTHER THAN PHYSICIAN (Please Print):

NAME:_____TITLE:_____EMPLOYER: _____

SECTION C: Narrative Description of Equipment and Cost

(1) Narrative description of all items, accessories and options ordered; (2) Supplier's charge; and (3) Medicare Fee Schedule Allowance for each item, accessory, and option. *(See instructions on back)*

SECTION D: Physician Attestation and Signature/Date

I certify that I am the physician identified in Section A of this form. I have received Sections A, B and C of the Certificate of Medical Necessity (including charges for items ordered). Any statement on my letterhead attached hereto, has been reviewed and signed by me. I certify that the medical necessity information in Section B is true, accurate and complete, to the best of my knowledge, and I understand that any falsification, omission, or concealment of material fact in that section may subject me to civil or criminal liability.

PHYSICIAN'S SIGNATURE_____DATE____/___/___(SIGNATURE AND DATE STAMPS ARE NOT ACCEPTABLE)

Form CMS-10269 (12/09)   1

Figure 1.2a: Certificate of Medical Necessity Page 1

Source: Centers for Medicare and Medicaid Services
Attribution: Centers for Medicare and Medicaid Services
License: Public Domain

INSTRUCTIONS FOR COMPLETING THE CERTIFICATE OF MEDICAL NECESSITY FOR POSITIVE AIRWAY PRESSURE (PAP) DEVICES FOR OBSTRUCTIVE SLEEP APNEA (CMS-10269)

SECTION A: (May be completed by the supplier)

CERTIFICATION TYPE/DATE: If this is an initial certification for this patient, indicate this by placing date (MM/DD/YY) needed initially in the space marked "INITIAL." If this is a revised certification (to be completed when the physician changes the order, based on the patient's changing clinical needs), indicate the initial date needed in the space marked "INITIAL," and also indicate the recertification date in the space marked "REVISED." If this is a recertification, indicate the initial date needed in the space marked "INITIAL," and also indicate the recertification date in the space marked "RECERTIFICATION." Whether submitting a REVISED or a RECERTIFIED CMN, be sure to always furnish the INITIAL date as well as the REVISED or RECERTIFICATION date.

PATIENT INFORMATION: Indicate the patient's name, permanent legal address, telephone number and his/her health insurance claim number (HICN) as it appears on his/her Medicare card and on the claim form.

SUPPLIER INFORMATION: Indicate the name of your company (supplier name), address and telephone number along with the National Provider Identification (NPI) number assigned to you by the National Supplier Clearinghouse (NSC).

PLACE OF SERVICE: Indicate the place in which the item is being used, i.e., patient's home is 12, skilled nursing facility (SNF) is 31, End Stage Renal Disease (ESRD) facility is 65, etc. Refer to the DME MAC supplier manual for a complete list.

FACILITY NAME: If the place of service is a facility, indicate the name and complete address of the facility.

HCPCS CODES: List all HCPCS procedure codes for items ordered that require a CMN. Procedure codes that do not require certification should not be listed on the CMN.

PATIENT DOB, HEIGHT, WEIGHT AND SEX: Indicate patient's date of birth (MM/DD/YY) and sex (male or female); height in inches and weight in pounds, if requested.

PHYSICIAN NAME, ADDRESS: Indicate the physician's name and complete mailing address.

NPI: Accurately indicate the ordering physician's National Provider Identification number (NPI).

PHYSICIAN'S TELEPHONE NO: Indicate the telephone number where the physician can be contacted (preferably where records would be accessible pertaining to this patient) if more information is needed.

SECTION B: (May not be completed by the supplier. While this section may be completed by a non-physician clinician, or a physician employee, it must be reviewed, and the CMN signed (in Section D) by the ordering physician.)

EST. LENGTH OF NEED: Indicate the estimated length of need (the length of time the physician expects the patient to require use of the ordered item) by filling in the appropriate number of months. If the physician expects that the patient will require the item for the duration of his/her life, then enter 99.

DIAGNOSIS CODES: In the first space, list the ICD9 code that represents the primary reason for ordering this item. List any additional ICD9 codes that would further describe the medical need for the item (up to 3 codes).

QUESTION SECTION: This section is used to gather clinical information to determine medical necessity. Answer each question which applies to the items ordered, checking "Y" for yes, "N" for no, or fill in the blank if other information is requested.

NAME OF PERSON ANSWERING SECTION B QUESTIONS: If a clinical professional other than the ordering physician (e.g., home health nurse, physical therapist, dietician) or a physician employee answers the questions of Section B, he/she must print his/her name, give his/her professional title and the name of his/her employer where indicated. If the physician is answering the questions, this space may be left blank.

SECTION C: (To be completed by the supplier)

NARRATIVE DESCRIPTION OF EQUIPMENT & COST: Supplier gives **(1)** a narrative description of the item(s) ordered, as well as all options, accessories, supplies and drugs; **(2)** the supplier's charge for each item, option, accessory, supply and drug; and **(3)** the Medicare fee schedule allowance for each item/option/accessory/supply/drug, if applicable.

SECTION D: (To be completed by the physician)

PHYSICIAN ATTESTATION: The physician's signature certifies **(1)** the CMN which he/she is reviewing includes Sections A, B, C and D; **(2)** the answers in Section B are correct; and **(3)** the self-identifying information in Section A is correct.

PHYSICIAN SIGNATURE AND DATE: After completion and/or review by the physician of Sections A, B and C, the physician must sign and date the CMN in Section D, verifying the Attestation appearing in this Section. The physician's signature also certifies the items ordered are medically necessary for this patient. Signature and date stamps are not acceptable.

According to the Paperwork Reduction Act of 1995, no persons are required to respond to a collection of information unless it displays a valid OMB control number. The valid OMB control number for this information collection is 0938-0679. The time required to complete this information collection is estimated to average 15 minutes per response, including the time to review instructions, search existing resources, gather the data needed, and complete and review the information collection. If you have any comments concerning the accuracy of the time estimate or suggestions for improving this form, please write to: CMS, 7500 Security Blvd., N2-14-26, Baltimore, Maryland 21244-1850.

Form CMS-10269 (12/09)   2

Figure 1.2b: Certificate of Medical Necessity Page 2

As you can see, many elements constitute compliance in healthcare settings. Lack of knowledge is not an acceptable excuse for noncompliance. It is every employee's responsibility to ensure they are compliant and/or report areas of noncompliance to be addressed immediately. Compliance programs provide guidance on regulatory issues and regulate the organization's activities to ensure compliance. The roles of compliance programs are threefold: prevention, detection, and correction. Healthcare employees need to be aware of their organization's policies and procedures to avoid disciplinary action, up to and including termination and/or incarceration.

1.8 SUMMARY

Health care in the U.S. has evolved over the past few centuries. As the U.S. continues to exert its global dominance in healthcare, organizations are tasked with complying with laws, regulations, policies, and procedures dictated by accrediting agencies. Compliance programs are one way healthcare organizations can ensure they are following these statutes and avoid being penalized.

1.9 DISCUSSION QUESTIONS

1. What is a compliance program?
2. Discuss the role of a compliance officer.
3. Discuss the benefits of a compliance program.
4. Who is responsible for ensuring a health care organization's compliance?
5. Based on the Joint Commission's list of unapproved abbreviations, indicate the appropriate category for each abbreviation: Unapproved or Discouraged

Abbreviation List	UNAPPROVED	DISCOURAGED
cc		
IU		
MSO4		
Trailing zero (X.o mg)		
> (greater than)		
@		
QD (qd)		
µg		
U (u)		

1.10 KEY TERM DEFINITIONS

1. Centers for Medicare and Medicaid Services (CMS) – the federal agency that runs the Medicare, Medicaid, and Children's Health Insurance Programs. CMS is a division of the Department of Health and Human Services (HHS).

2. Chief Executive Officer (CEO) – the highest-ranking person in a company or other institution who is ultimately responsible for making managerial decisions.

3. Compliance Officer – an individual who ensures that a company complies with its outside regulatory and legal requirements as well as internal policies and bylaws.

4. Healthcare compliance – the process of following rules, regulations, and laws that relate to healthcare practices.

5. Office of Inspector General (OIG) – the federal agency responsible for ensuring that the health care industry complies with fraud and abuse laws. OIG also seeks to educate the public about fraudulent schemes so that individuals can protect themselves and report suspicious activities.

6. Third-Party Payer – an entity (other than the patient or the health care provider) that reimburses and manages healthcare expenses.

1.11 REFERENCES

Agency for Healthcare Research and Quality. (2017). Estimating the additional hospital inpatient cost and mortality associated with selected hospital-acquired conditions. Retrieved from https://www.ahrq.gov/hai/pfp/haccost2017-results.html

Atherton, J. (2011). Development of the electronic health record. *AMA Journal of Ethics, Virtual Mentor, 13*(3):186-189. doi: 10.1001/virtualmentor.2011.13.3.mhst1-1103.

Blair, P.L. (2012). Lateral violence in nursing. *Journal of Emergency Nursing, 38*, 1-4. doi: 10.1016/j.jen.2011.12.006

Department of Justice. (2011). The False Claims Act: A Primer. Retrieved from https://www.justice.gov/sites/default/files/civil/legacy/2011/04/22/C-FRAUDS_FCA_Primer.pdf

Ditmer, D. (2010). A safe environment for nurses and patients: Halting horizontal violence. *Journal of Nursing Regulation, 1*(3), 9-14.

Hartunian, R.S., Wolff, J.C., & Seigel, R. (2017, November). Fraud and abuse 2017: Understanding trends and avoiding actions. Retrieved from https://www.manatt.com/Insights/Newsletters/Health-Update/Fraud-and-Abuse-2017-Understanding-Trends-and-Avoi?utm_source=healthupdatenewsletter&utm_medium=email&utm_campaign=healthupdate_11.21.17#Article1

Hartunian, R.S., Wolff, J.C., & Seigel, R. (2018, January). *The eight key elements of*

effective compliance programs. Retrieved from https://www.manatt.com/Insights/
Newsletters/Health-Update/The-Eight-Key-Elements-of-Effective-Compliance-Pro

James, J.T. (2013). A new, evidence-based estimate of patient harms associated
with hospital care. *Journal of Patient Safety, 9*(3):122-8. doi: 10.1097/
PTS.0b013e3182948a69

National Academy of Sciences. (2017). *Global health and the future role of
the United States: A consensus study report of the National Academies of
Sciences•Engineering•Medicine.* Washington, DC: The National Academies Press.

Neilsen, M., & Einarsen, S. (2012). Outcomes of exposure to workplace bullying: A
meta-analytic review. *Work & Stress: An International Journal of Work, Health &
Organisations, 26*, 309-332.

Office of Inspector General. (2011). *Health care fraud prevention and enforcement
action team (HEAT) provider compliance training* [Presentation]. Washington, DC:
Office of the Inspector General.

Pettinger, T. (2019). Advantages of capitalism. Retrieved from www.economicshelp.org

Probasco, J. (2019). Why do healthcare costs keep rising? Retrieved from www.
investopedia.com

Rodziewicz, T.L., & Hipskind, J.E. (2019). Medical Error Prevention. StatPearls
Publishing LLC.

Safian, S.C. (2009). *Essentials of Health Care Compliance.* Clifton Park, NY: Delmar,
Cengage Learning.

The Joint Commission. (2019). Official "Do Not Use" List. Retrieved from https://www.
jointcommission.org/facts_about_do_not_use_list/

Thorpe, K. (2011, May 25). Medical advancements: Who is leading the world? *HuffPost
News.* Retrieved September 27, 2019 from HuffPost.com

United States. Department of Justice. (2018). *National health care fraud takedown
results in charges against 601 individuals responsible for over $2 billion in
fraud losses.* Retrieved from https://www.justice.gov/opa/pr/national-health-
care-fraud-takedown-results-charges-against-601-individuals-responsible-
over#:~:text=Azar%20III%2C%20announced%20today%20the,than%20%242%20
billion%20in%20false

2 Ethics and Law

2.1 LEARNING OBJECTIVES

1. Demonstrate a comprehensive overview of health law.
2. Compare and contrast the differences between legal and ethical issues in healthcare.
3. Describe the role of healthcare enforcement agencies in legal and ethical situations.
4. Identify the major healthcare laws and regulations that pertain to fraud and abuse.

2.2 INTRODUCTION

Ethics and law are important topics to consider when thinking about healthcare compliance. While compliance means following the law, ethics means doing the right thing even without a law. Many federal and state agencies enforce healthcare laws and regulations to ensure compliance. Healthcare providers and organizations must be knowledgeable of industry laws and regulations in order to ensure best practice and avoid prosecution. In addition, licensing agencies for healthcare professionals require that professionals follow a code of ethical conduct. This chapter will explore the major healthcare laws, enforcement agencies, and issues surrounding ethical behavior relative to compliance in healthcare organizations.

2.3 KEY TERMS

- Ethics
- Laws
- Fraud
- Abuse

- Healthcare Laws
- Enforcement Agencies

2.4 ETHICAL CHALLENGES IN HEALTHCARE

Ethics can be defined as the moral principles and set of values that an individual holds in regards to what is right and what is wrong (Daft, 2016). Four important principles of ethics guide our actions in healthcare: beneficence, nonmaleficence, justice, and respect for others. Beneficence refers to a healthcare provider's responsibility to do what is in the best interest of others (Olden, 2015). Healthcare organizations are ethically responsible for doing all they can to alleviate pain and suffering associated with health care conditions (Shi & Singh, 2015). Nonmaleficence refers to healthcare providers' responsibility to do no harm to patients. Since many health care treatments may present risks to patients, nonmaleficence requires that the benefits outweigh the risks of medical treatment (Shi & Singh, 2015). The principle of justice refers to fairness and equality, requiring that there be no discrimination in the delivery of healthcare services (Shi & Singh, 2015). The principle of respect for others requires that healthcare providers show respect for the autonomy, privacy, rights, and interests of patients. This means providing patients with all necessary information required for their making an informed decision, and allowing patients to make such decisions regarding their own care without coercion, and obtaining consent for treatment (Shi & Singh, 2015). Four key aspects of medical ethics are included within the principle of respect for persons: autonomy, truth-telling, confidentiality, and fidelity. Autonomy refers to individuals having the right to make their own decisions regarding their care. Truth-telling refers to providers being honest with patients. Confidentiality refers to keeping patient information private (Buchbinder & Shanks, 2017). Fidelity refers to providers performing their duties, keeping their word, and keeping promises (Shi & Singh, 2015).

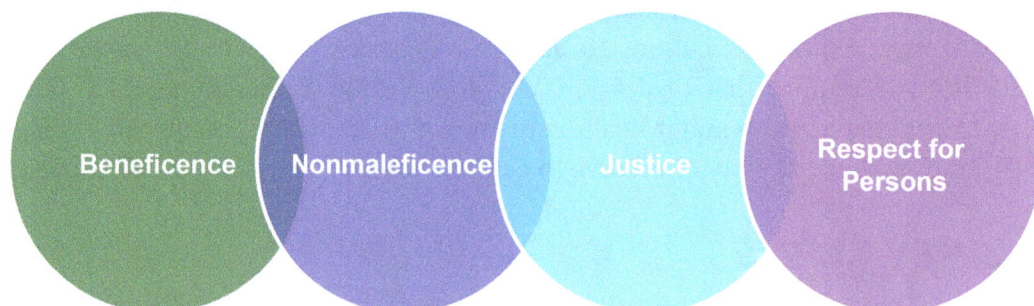

Figure 2.1: Four Principles of Ethics

Source: Original Work
Attribution: Lesley Clack
License: CC BY-SA 4.0

Healthcare providers are often faced with situations surrounding ethical behavior. Ethically challenging situations in healthcare include abortion, artificial prolongation of life, and physician-assisted suicide (Shi & Singh, 2017). These types of situations can present a conflict of interest for the provider. A conflict of interest is a situation in which an individual's self-interest interferes with that individual's obligation to another person or organization (Olden, 2015). These situations often conflict with a provider's own morals and values and can cause them immense distress when determining the most ethical course of action. An individual's source of ethics comes from a variety of sources, such as their own personal experiences, their organization, and their profession. While many healthcare organizations have a code of ethics that employees must follow, healthcare professionals must also follow the code of ethics of their professional association (Table 1).

Professional Association	Provider Type	Link to Code of Ethics
American Medical Association (AMA)	Physician	https://www.ama-assn.org/delivering-care/ethics/code-medical-ethics-overview
American Nurses Association (ANA)	Nurse	https://www.nursingworld.org/~4aef79/globalassets/docs/ana/ethics/anastatement-ethicshumanrights-january2017.pdf
American College of Healthcare Executives (ACHE)	Healthcare Managers, Administrators, and Executives	https://www.ache.org/-/media/ache/ethics/code_of_ethics_web.pdf?la=en&hash=F8D67234C06C333793BB58402D73741A4ACE3D9D

Table 2.1: Code of Ethics for Healthcare Professional Associations

Source: Original Work
Attribution: Lesley Clack
License: CC BY-SA 4.0

Real-Life Case: Unethical Behavior

In 2014, Dr. Joseph Darrow, Jr., an orthopedic surgeon, engaged in a sexual relationship with a patient concurrent with, or immediately following, the physician-patient relationship and married the patient. The Iowa Board of Medicine concluded that Dr. Darrow violated the licensing board's ethical code of conduct which states that physicians are not allowed to have a sexual relationship with patients. The case was settled, and the physician agreed to pay a $5,000 civil penalty (Iowa Board of Medicine, 2014).

Real-Life Case: Unethical Behavior

In 2016, a Charleston, WV physician, Dr. Iraj Derakhshan, was charged with violating reporting requirements mandated by federal drug laws for dispensing controlled substances. Dr. Derakhshan admitted that a patient returned unused fentanyl, and he illegally dispensed it to another patient. The physician also admitted he was never authorized to dispense controlled substances. Dr. Derakhshan permanently surrendered his license for dispensing controlled substances and was ordered to pay a fine of $10,000.

2.5 LEGAL CONSIDERATIONS

Healthcare laws regulate the provision of healthcare services and govern the relationship between those who provide care and those who receive care. Laws are essential rules of conduct that help us determine both our and others' actions (Buchbinder & Shanks, 2017). Laws are standards a society considers to be the minimum principles necessary to keep that society functioning (Judson & Harrison, 2019). An unethical act is not necessarily illegal, but an illegal act by a healthcare provider is always unethical (Judson & Harrison, 2019). Federal health agencies design healthcare laws with the goal of protecting the interests and well-being of the public. Congress provides oversight of healthcare laws and regulations. And the Department of Health and Human Services (HHS) provides general oversight in regards to health issues and concerns. The mission of HHS is to "enhance and protect the health and well-being of all Americans;" this is achieved by "providing for effective health and human services and fostering advances in medicine, public health, and social services" (HHS, 2019). Table 2 includes a list of some of the most influential healthcare laws.

Law	Year Passed	Description
The Social Security Act of 1935	1935	The Social Security Act of 1935 was enacted by Congress and signed into law by President Franklin D. Roosevelt. This act established the Social Security program, an old-age program funded by payroll taxes, and insurance against unemployment.
Medicare	1965	Medicare was enacted by Congress and signed into law by President Johnson under the Social Security Amendments of 1965. The Medicare program was designed to provide health care coverage for individuals over the age of 65. Since its inception, Medicare has been expanded to add coverage for individuals with disabilities and end-stage renal diseases. Medicare is administered by the Centers for Medicare and Medicaid Services (CMS).
Medicaid	1965	Medicaid was established by adding Title XIX to the Social Security Act. Medicaid was designed to provide health care coverage for individuals receiving public assistance, such as low-income elderly, the blind, or the disabled. Medicaid has since been expanded and now includes low-income children and parents, pregnant women, the disabled, and impoverished adults. Medicaid is administered by the states and receives a combination of state and federal funding.
Children's Health Insurance Program (CHIP)	1997	CHIP is administered by CMS. CHIP was designed to provide coverage for children who are not eligible for Medicaid but whose parents are unable to afford private insurance coverage. CHIP is a state-administered program, with each state setting their own eligibility requirements.

Health Insurance Portability and Accountability Act of 1996 (HIPAA)	1996	HIPAA was established to create guidelines regarding how personally identifiable information should be maintained by healthcare organizations and to set limitations on healthcare insurance coverage. HIPAA was enacted by Congress and signed into law by President Clinton.
HIPAA Privacy Rule	2003	The goal of the HIPAA Privacy Rule is to ensure that an individual's health information is properly protected while not inhibiting the flow of health information needed for that individual to receive high quality care.
HIPAA Security Rule	2005	The HIPAA Security Rule establishes national standards for protecting an individual's electronic personal health information and how it is created, received, used, or maintained.
Patient Safety and Quality Improvement Act of 2005 (PSQIA)	2005	PSQIA establishes a voluntary reporting system which is designed to enhance the data available to assess and resolve patient safety and health care quality issues. PSQIA authorizes HHS to impose civil money penalties for violations of patient safety and confidentiality.
Patient Protection and Affordable Care Act (PPACA)	2010	PPACA is a federal statute that was enacted by Congress and signed into law by President Obama. The goal of PPACA was to provide a regulatory overhaul and expansion of coverage. The most well-known provision of the PPACA was the implementation of an individual mandate that required individuals to have health insurance coverage or they would have to pay a penalty on their taxes.

OVERVIEW OF HEALTHCARE COMPLIANCE

Hospital Readmissions Reduction Program (HRRP)	2012	The HRRP is a Medicare value-based purchasing program that reduces payments to hospitals with excess readmissions. The rate of readmission is a quality indicator; thus, this program seeks to improve the quality of health care for Americans.
Tax Cuts and Jobs Act of 2017	2017	In regards to its impact on healthcare, this legislation, enacted under the Trump administration, repealed the individual mandate of the PPACA. This repeal takes effect in 2019.

Table 2.2: Influential Healthcare Laws

Source: Original Work
Attribution: Lesley Clack
License: CC BY-SA 4.0

Real-Life Example: HIPAA Violation

In September 2015, Memorial Hermann Health System (MHHS), a hospital health system serving the Houston, Texas area provided an unauthorized disclosure of protected health information, which is in violation of the HIPAA Privacy Rule. A patient that visited an MHHS clinic presented a fraudulent identification card to hospital staff. The fraudulent ID card was identified by hospital staff which notified law enforcement, and the patient was arrested. The hospital disclosed the name of the patient to law enforcement, which is allowable under HIPAA. However, the hospital then issued a press release about the incident, disclosing the patient's name in the title of the press release. Releasing the patient's name to the media without permission was an impermissible disclosure of protected health information. A complaint was filed with the Office of Civil Rights, and MHHS agreed to a settlement of $2.4 million, in addition to agreeing to adopt a corrective action plan that requires policies and procedures to be updated and training staff to prevent further impermissible disclosures of protected health information.

2.6 ENFORCEMENT

As noted above, a variety of different agencies regulate and govern healthcare in the U.S. Under Title XXVII of the Public Health Service Act (PHS Act), states are given the responsibility of exercising primary enforcement over health insurers to ensure they comply with health insurance market forms (CMS, Compliance and Enforcement, 2019). The HHS Office for Civil Rights holds the responsibility for enforcing the HIPAA Privacy and Security Rules (HHS, HIPAA Enforcement, 2019). Key healthcare enforcement agencies and their responsibilities are listed in Table 3.

Agency	Description
Agency for Healthcare Research and Quality (AHRQ)	The primary function of AHRQ is to support research designed to improve health care quality and outcomes, reduce costs, address patient safety and medical errors, and improve access to health care.
Agency for Toxic Substances and Disease Registry (ATSDR)	The mission of ATSDR is to prevent exposure and adverse human health effects and diminished quality of life associated with exposure to hazardous substances from waste sites, unplanned releases, and other sources of pollution present in the environment.
Centers for Disease Control (CDC)	The mission of the CDC is to promote health and quality of life by preventing and controlling disease, injury, and disability. The CDC works with national and international partners to monitor health, detect and investigate health problems, conduct research to enhance prevention, develop and advocate sound public health policies, implement prevention strategies, promote healthy behaviors, foster safe and healthful environments, and provide leadership and training.
Department of Health and Human Services Office for Civil Rights (OCR)	OCR is responsible for enforcing HIPAA rules and regulations.
Food and Drug Administration (FDA)	The FDA ensures the safety of foods and cosmetics and the safety and efficacy of pharmaceuticals, biological products, and medical devices. Its employees monitor the manufacture, import, transport, storage, and sale of about $1 trillion worth of products each year.
Health Resources and Services Administration (HRSA)	The HRSA directs national health programs that improve the nation's health by assuring equitable access to comprehensive, quality health care for all. HRSA also works to improve and extend life for people living with HIV/ AIDS, provide primary health care to medically underserved people, serve women and children through state programs, and train a health workforce that is both diverse and motivated to work in underserved communities.

Centers for Medicare and Medicaid Services (CMS)	CMS administers the Medicare and Medicaid programs, in addition to other major programs such as the State Children's Health Insurance Program (SCHIP); the Medicare Prescription Drug, Improvement, and Modernization Act (MMA); and the Health Insurance Portability and Accountability Act (HIPAA). The mission of CMS is to ensure healthcare security for its beneficiaries.
Indian Health Services (IHS)	IHS provides comprehensive healthcare services, including preventive, curative, rehabilitative, and environmental care for American Indians and Alaska Natives who belong to more than 550 federally recognized tribes in 35 states.
National Institutes of Health (NIH)	NIH, the Nation's medical research agency, is composed of 27 Institutes and Centers. NIH provides leadership and financial support to researchers in every state, and throughout the world, helping to lead the way toward important medical discoveries that improve people's health and save lives.
Office of the National Coordinator for Health IT (ONC)	ONC is responsible for coordinating nationwide efforts to implement and use health information technology. This includes implementation of initiatives, such as electronic health record (EHR) adoption.
Substance Abuse and Mental Health Services Administration (SAMHSA)	SAMHSA works to improve the quality and availability of prevention, treatment, and rehabilitative services in order to reduce illness, death, disability, and cost to society resulting from substance abuse and mental illnesses.

Table 2.3: Key Healthcare Enforcement Agencies (USPHS, 2019)

Source: Original Work
Attribution: Lesley Clack
License: CC BY-SA 4.0

2.7 FRAUD AND ABUSE

Fraud and abuse have always been areas of concern in healthcare. In particular, Medicare and Medicaid experience a high prevalence of fraud and abuse (Shi & Singh, 2017). Fraud has been defined as "an intentional act of deception," while abuse has been defined as "improper acts that are unintentional but inconsistent with standard practices" (Buchbinder & Shanks, 2017, p. 442). Abuse is considered to be an unintentional mistreatment, while fraud constitutes an intentional act. Examples of fraud and abuse in healthcare include billing for services not provided, billing for services that are not medically necessary, submitting duplicate bills, and improperly using codes to receive higher reimbursement (Buchbinder & Shanks, 2017). Several laws and regulations have been established to specifically address fraud and abuse (Table 4).

Law	Year Passed	Description	Penalties
False Claims Act	1863	The False Claims Act imposes liability on any person who knowingly submits or causes the submission of false or fraudulent claims for payment or approval.	No less than $5,000 or more than $10,000, plus potential damages, for each false claim filed.
Anti-Kickback Statute	1972	The Anti-Kickback Statute prohibits providers of services covered by a Federal healthcare program from receiving anything of value in order to induce or reward patient referrals.	Up to $25,000 per violation, felony conviction punishable by imprisonment up to 5 years, or both, as well as possible exclusion from participation in Federal Healthcare Programs.
Stark Law	1989	The Stark Law prohibits the referral of Medicare and Medicaid beneficiaries by a physician to an entity in which the physician has a financial relationship.	Up to $15,000 for each claim submitted in violation of the statute.
Exclusion Provisions	1999	Under Section 1128 of the Social Security Act, the HHS Office of Inspector General (OIG) has authority to exclude individuals from participating in federal health care programs for various reasons, such as program-related crimes, convictions related to patient abuse, felony convictions related to health care fraud, and felony convictions related to controlled substances.	Up to $10,000 per item or service claimed while excluded. HHS may also impose an assessment of up to three times the amount claimed.
Civil Monetary Penalties Law	2001	The Civil Monetary Penalties Law, Section 1128A of the Social Security Act, authorizes HHS-OIG to impose civil penalties for violations of the Anti-Kickback Statute and other related violations.	Range from $10,000 to $50,000 per violation.

Table 2.4: Laws & Regulations Related to Fraud & Abuse

Source: Original Work
Attribution: Lesley Clack
Source: CC BY-SA 4.0

> **Real-Life Example: False Claims Act, Stark Law, and Anti-Kickback Statute Violation**
>
> Amedisys, one of the country's largest providers of home health services, based in Baton Rouge, Louisiana, and its affiliates agreed to pay $150 million to resolve allegations brought under the False Claims Act, Stark Law and the Anti-Kickback Statute. The lawsuit filed against Amedisys was brought under the *qui tam*, or whistle-blower, provision of the False Claims Act by former employees of the company. The lawsuit alleged Amedisys submitted improper claims to Medicare for reimbursement from 2008 to 2010 for therapy and nursing services that were medically unnecessary or provided to patients who were not homebound. The lawsuit also alleged the company engaged in improper financial relationships with referring physicians.

2.8 IMPLICATIONS FOR COMPLIANCE

The many healthcare codes of ethics, laws, and regulations we've discussed serve as a source of compliance in healthcare. OIG recommends that organizations adopt a corporate compliance plan which assist in ensuring the organization complies with all laws and regulations and seeks to reduce risk of errors or omission (Buchbinder & Shanks, 2017). The OIG provides a list of elements that are considered essential for any compliance program (OIG, 2017):

- Element 1: Standards, Policies, and Procedures
- Element 2: Compliance Program Administration
- Element 3: Screening and Evaluation of Employees, Physicians, Vendors and other Agents
- Element 4: Communication, Education, and Training on Compliance Issues
- Element 5: Monitoring, Auditing, and Internal Reporting Systems
- Element 6: Discipline for Non-Compliance
- Element 7: Investigations and Remedial Measures

Healthcare organizations must ensure compliance with all laws and regulations, and a corporate compliance program is instrumental in meeting this objective.

2.9 SUMMARY

Governance of healthcare delivery comes from a wide variety of sources, such as ethical codes of conduct, healthcare laws and regulations, and enforcement agencies. Protecting patients is the utmost concern, which is one of the reasons that healthcare is such a highly regulated industry. With the healthcare landscape constantly changing, and new laws and regulations continually added over time, it is vital that healthcare providers and organizations stay up to date. Good corporate compliance is essential when dealing with law and ethics in the healthcare industry.

2.10 DISCUSSION QUESTIONS

1. Find a recent case in the media regarding the violation of a healthcare law. Which law is addressed in the case? What were the main issues in the case? Did the plaintiff win their case? Why or why not?

2. Think of an example of unethical behavior that you have heard of or have observed in healthcare. Which of the four ethical principles were violated in this situation? If you were a manager, how would you deal with this behavior? Is the behavior only unethical, or is it also illegal? If so, which healthcare law is also violated in the situation?

3. An administrator at the hospital you work for has ordered all physicians to use codes with the highest reimbursement rates. A physician in the emergency room has billed for services that were not provided. Is this fraud or abuse? What should the hospital do?

4. You are an administrator for a home health agency. Write a brief compliance plan using the OIG's seven essential elements for a compliance plan.

2.11 KEY TERM DEFINITIONS

1. Ethics—the moral principles and set of values that an individual holds in regards to what is right and what is wrong.

2. Laws—essential rules of conduct that help us determine our actions and others' actions and are considered to be the minimum principles necessary to keep society functioning.

3. Fraud—an intentional act of deception.

4. Abuse—improper acts that are unintentional but inconsistent with standard practices.

5. Healthcare Laws—regulate the provision of healthcare services and govern the relationship between those who provide care and those who receive care.

6. Enforcement Agencies—agencies that regulate and govern health care in the U.S.

2.12 REFERENCES

Buchbinder, S.B. & Shanks, N.H. (2017). *Introduction to Health Care Management, 3*rd *edition.*

Burlington, MA: Jones & Bartlett Learning.

Centers for Medicare and Medicaid Services. (2019). Compliance and Enforcement. Retrieved from https://www.cms.gov/cciio/programs-and-initiatives/health-insurance-market-reforms/compliance.html

Daft, R.L. (2016). *Organization Theory and Design, 12*th *edition*. Boston, MA: Cengage Learning.

Department of Health and Human Services (HHS). (2019). About HHS. Retrieved from https://www.hhs.gov/about/index.html

Department of Health and Human Services (HHS). (2019). HIPAA Enforcement. Retrieved from https://www.hhs.gov/hipaa/for-professionals/compliance-enforcement/index.html

Iowa Board of Medicine. (2014). In the Matter of Statement Charges Against Joseph C. Darrow, Jr., M.D., Respondent. Retrieved from https://medicalboard.iowa.gov/sites/default/files/documents/2018/04/darrowjosephc.jr_.m.d.-02-2014-468.pdf

Judson, K. & Harrison, C. (2019). *Law & Ethics for Health Professions, 8*th *edition*. New York, NY: McGraw-Hill Education.

Measuring Compliance Program Effectiveness: A Resource Guide. Retrieved from https://oig.hhs.gov/compliance/101/files/HCCA-OIG-Resource-Guide.pdf

Office of the Inspector General (OIG), Department of Health and Human Services. (2017).

Olden, P.C. (2015). *Management of Healthcare Organizations: An Introduction*. Chicago, IL: Health Administration Press.

Shi, L. & Singh, D.A. (2015). *Delivering Health Care in America: A Systems Approach*. Burlington, MA: Jones & Bartlett Learning.

Shi, L. & Singh, D.A. (2017). *Essentials of the U.S. Health Care System, 4*th *edition*. Burlington, MA: Jones & Bartlett Learning.

US Public Health Service (USPHS). (2019). HHS Offices and Agencies. Retrieved from https://www.usphs.gov/aboutus/agencies/hhs.aspx

3 Health Insurance & Reimbursement

3.1 LEARNING OBJECTIVES

1. Identify innovative new approaches to the payer/provider model.
2. Differentiate between the types of health insurance.
3. Analyze the laws that govern health insurance & reimbursement practices.
4. Describe the effects of noncompliance with reimbursement practices.

3.2 INTRODUCTION

Various United States insurance plans include government based and private payers. When these payers fail to adhere to reporting requirements for reimbursement, results can include losses in revenue, penalties, fines, and a revocation of business licenses. This chapter will discuss the types of insurance plans currently available, innovative approaches to the established payer/ provider model, and standard reimbursement practices. The laws that govern health insurance and reimbursement practices will be examined and the effects of noncompliance reviewed.

3.3 KEY TERMS

- Accountable Care Organizations (ACOs)
- Electronic Health Record (EHR)
- Federal Poverty Level (FPL)
- Fee-for-service (FFS)
- Health Maintenance Organization (HMO)
- Preferred Provider Organizations (PPO)
- Primary Care Physician (PCP)

3.4 HISTORICAL EVOLUTION OF PAYER MODELS

Prior to the 1900s, health insurance as we know it today did not exist in the United States. However, employers such as railroad companies did develop "hospital associations" where employees could receive health care from physicians who were employed by the railroad company (Kongstvedt, 2020). Trade unions also offered employees they represented financial protection in case they became ill or injured. Kaiser, one of today's most well-known names in health care and insurance, initially began as a construction company that offered coverage for their employees (this plan would later become known as the Kaiser Health Plan).

By the mid 1800's, several companies offered commercial and/or group health insurance programs. However, these companies were not financially successful because they attracted large numbers of sick individuals and did not charge premiums sufficient to cover their expenses. Although the insurance industry was beginning to expand, the policies offered were not the same as modern day health insurance.

Prior to World War II (WWII), only 10% of patients had any type of health benefits, thus most patients paid for any health services they received out of pocket (Kongstvedt, 2020). By the mid-1950s, however, almost 70% of patients had health benefits. Several reasons account for this increase in health coverage, such as the following:

- Individuals were driven to obtain health benefits to allow for improved and affordable health care;
- Physicians sought ways to generate steady, reliable revenue;
- Employers offered health benefits as a means to recruit and retain employees;
- Lending agencies encouraged their clients to obtain health benefits to reduce the number of foreclosures that occurred due to health-related personal bankruptcies (Kongstvedt, 2020).

In addition to these incentives, one additional factor influenced Americans to obtain health benefits. Due to the scarcity of physical resources and available workforce after WWII, the U.S. government passed the 1942 Stabilization Act. The act prevented employers from paying higher wages to attract workers. However, the act did allow for certain employer contributions (including health benefits) to be non-taxable. As a result, workers were motivated to obtain employer-based health benefits to offset their taxable income.

Two health benefit models were available during this time: health maintenance organizations (HMOs) and Blue Cross and Blue Shield plans. HMOs charge a set fee per person/enrollee who must receive care from one of the HMO's facilities and providers (commonly referred to as in-network facilities and providers). Blue Cross and Blue Shield (BC/BS) plans contracted with healthcare facilities and providers in the community and allowed their members to obtain care at any of the covered sites. However, BC/BS plans were prepaid benefits, not health insurance as we know it today. These two models were the precursors of today's HMOs and Preferred Provider Organizations (PPOs).

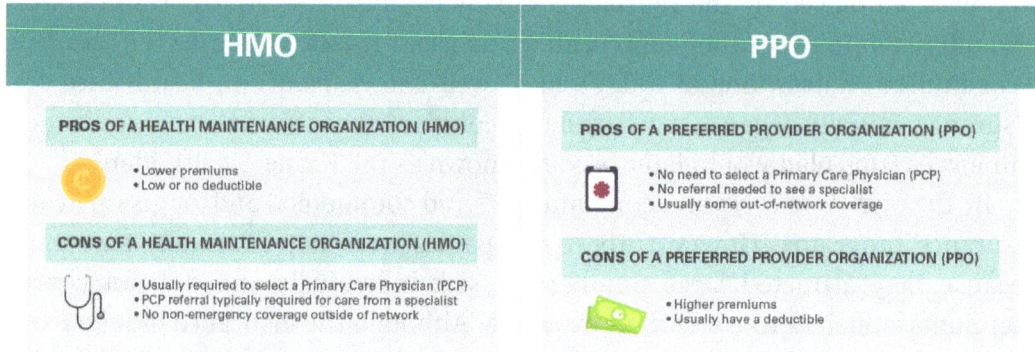

Figure 3.1: HMO & PPO Comparison Chart

Source: Medical Mutual of Ohio ®

Attribution: Medical Mutual of Ohio ®

License: © Medical Mutual of Ohio ®. Used with permission.

HMOs later transformed their structure to one referred to as an independent practice association (IPA) (Kongstvedt, 2020). In contrast to the previous structure, which was composed of HMOs with their own dedicated medical staff and facilities, the newly formed IPAs included contracts with independent physicians or with organizations who contract with physicians.

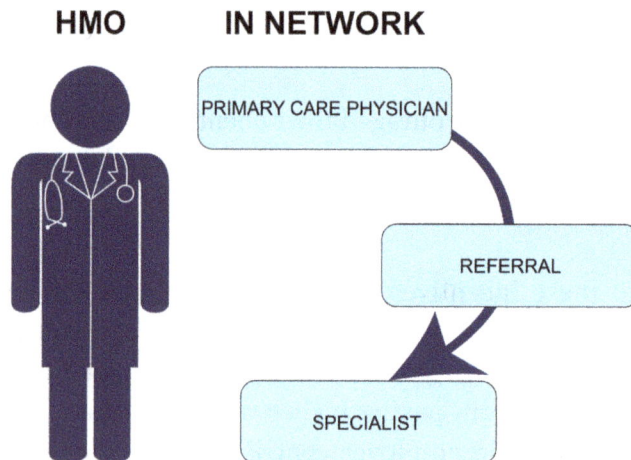

Figure 3.2: HMO Flowchart

Source: Original Work

Attribution: Corey Parson

License: CC BY-SA 4.0

Medicare was established in 1965 by Title XVIII of the Social Security Act, beginning with Medicare Part A which covers hospital services, and Medicare Part B which covers physicians' services (Klees, Wolfe, & Curtis, 2009). Part A was funded through taxes on earned income while Part B was funded through premiums and general revenues (Kongstvedt, 2020). Medicare was initially offered to those individuals who were age 65 or over. However, additional groups were later added, including individuals who are:

- Entitled to Social Security or Railroad Retirement disability for at least 24 months;
- Diagnosed with certain illnesses such as end-stage renal disease (ESRD);
- Otherwise not eligible but elect to pay a premium.

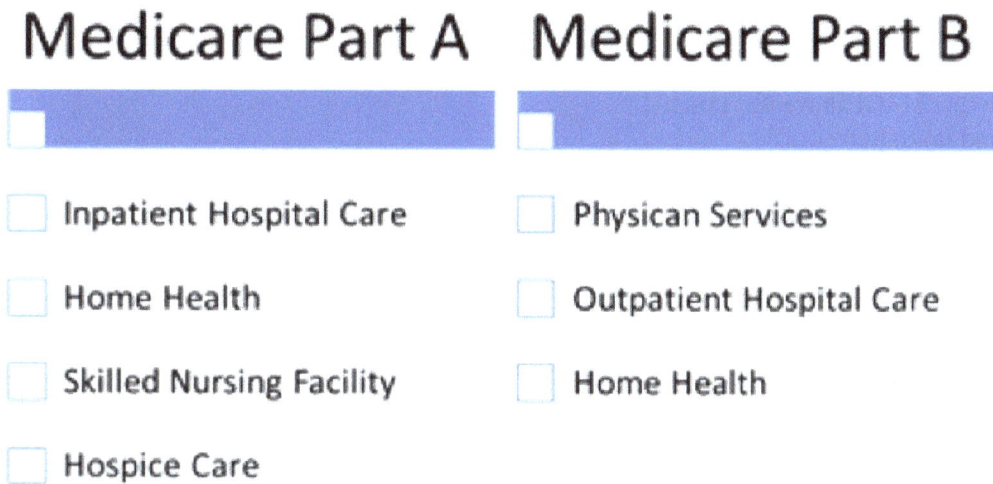

Medicare Part A   Medicare Part B

- Inpatient Hospital Care
- Home Health
- Skilled Nursing Facility
- Hospice Care

- Physican Services
- Outpatient Hospital Care
- Home Health

Figure 3.3: Medicare Parts A & B Coverage

Source: Original Work
Attribution: Larecia Gill
License: CC BY-SA 4.0

In 1997, the Balanced Budget Act (BBA) established the Medicare+Choice program, otherwise referred to as Medicare Part C or the Medicare Advantage Program. This program was modified and renamed in 2003 as the Medicare Prescription Drug, Improvement, and Modernization Act (MMA) which expanded recipients' options in private-sector health plans (Klees, Wolfe, & Curtis, 2009). The MMA also added Medicare Part D, which provides prescription drug coverage.

As the program has continued, there have been changes to the coverage, premium, and age of eligibility. For example, beneficiaries with higher incomes pay a higher premium for Part B and prescription drug coverage (Social Security Administration, 2019). The monthly Medicare Part B premiums for 2019 are listed in table 3.1:

Modified Adjusted Gross Income (MAGI)	Part B Monthly Premium Amount	Prescription Drug Coverage Monthly Premium Amount
Individuals with a MAGI of $85,000 or less, married couples with a MAGI of $170,000 or less	2019 standard premium = $135.50	Your plan premium
Individuals with a MAGI above $85,000 and up to $107,000, married couples with a MAGI above $170,000 and up to $214,000	Standard premium + $54.10	Your plan premium + $12.40
Individuals with a MAGI above $107,000 and up to $133,500, married couples with a MAGI above $214,000 and up to $267,000	Standard premium + $135.40	Your plan premium + $31.90
Individuals with a MAGI above $133,500 and up to $160,000, married couples with a MAGI above $267,000 and up to $320,000	Standard premium + $216.70	Your plan premium + $51.40
Individuals with a MAGI above $160,000 and up to $500,000, married couples with a MAGI above $320,000 and up to $750,000	Standard premium + $297.90	Your plan premium + $70.90
Individuals with a MAGI equal to or above $500,000, married couples with a MAGI equal to or above $750,000	Standard premium + $325.00	Your plan premium + $77.40

Table 3.1: The standard Part B premium for 2019 is $135.50. If you're single and filed an individual tax return, or married and filed a joint tax return, the following applies to you:

Source: Social Security Administration
Attribution: Social Security Administration
License: Public Domain

Title XIX of the Social Security Act established Medicaid, which is a program jointly funded by the federal and state governments to provide medical care for individuals with low incomes (Klees, Wolfe, & Curtis, 2009). Within federal guidelines, each state establishes eligibility criteria, authorized services, and reimbursement rates. Therefore, individuals who may qualify for Medicaid benefits in one state may not be eligible in other states. Although each state determines the eligibility criteria, all must include the following requirements for applicants:

- Be a resident of the state for which they are applying for coverage;

- Be a citizen of the United States or a member of certain qualified non-citizen groups such as lawful permanent residents;
- Meet set modified adjusted gross income (MAGI) levels;
- Include children who are covered by the adoption assistance agreement under Title IV-E of the Social Security Act.

States may opt to include individuals deemed "medically needy" whose financial status is too high to qualify for Medicaid (Centers for Medicare & Medicaid Services, 2019, Medicaid Eligibility).

Title XXI of the Social Security Act established the Children's Health Insurance Program (CHIP; formerly referred to as State Children's Health Insurance Program or SCHIP). This program provides funding for health coverage for children who are from low-income households but do not qualify for Medicaid. These children would generally be uninsured without the availability of CHIP. Each state establishes eligibility criteria for CHIP (see figure 3.4).

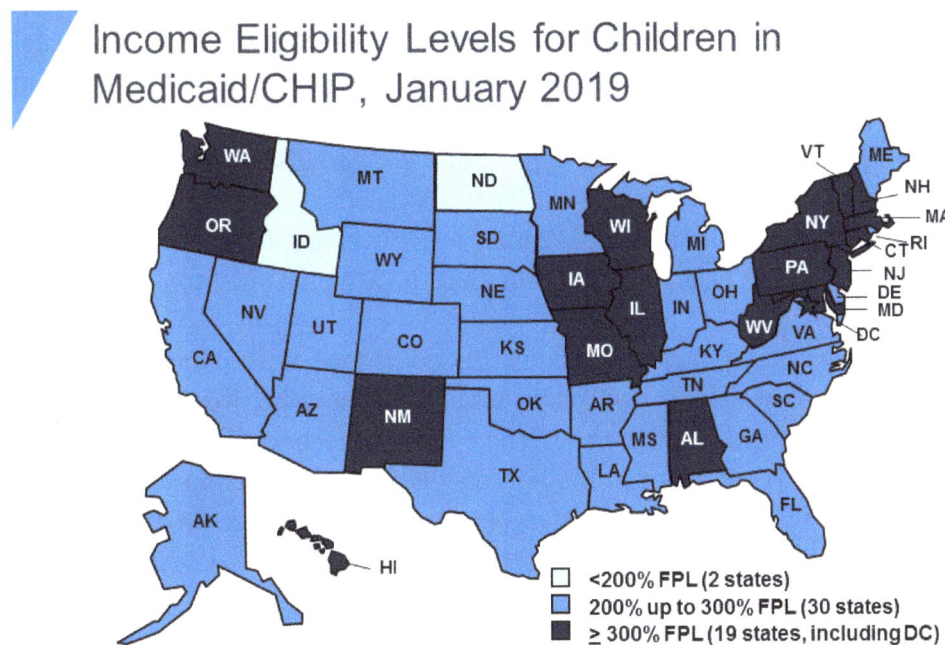

Income Eligibility Levels for Children in Medicaid/CHIP, January 2019

☐ <200% FPL (2 states)
■ 200% up to 300% FPL (30 states)
■ ≥ 300% FPL (19 states, including DC)

NOTE: Eligibility levels are based on 2019 federal poverty levels (FPLs) for a family of three. In 2019, the FPL was $21,330 for a family of three. Thresholds include the standard five percentage point of the FPL disregard.
SOURCE: Based on results from a national survey conducted by the Kaiser Family Foundation and the Georgetown University Center for Children and Families, 2019.

KFF

Figure 3.4: Income Eligibility Levels for Children in Medicaid/CHIP, January 2019

Source: Kaiser Family Foundation
Attribution: Kaiser Family Foundation
License: © Kaiser Family Foundation. Used with permission.

3.5 TYPES OF INSURANCE

Three distinct markets offer health insurance plans: coverage purchased by individuals, group coverage offered by employers and paid for by employer and employee premiums, and governmental entitlement programs (Kongstvedt, 2020). Medicare and Medicaid are both examples of government payer insurance plans. In general, there are two major types of *private* payer insurance in the U.S.: traditional (indemnity) and managed care.

3.5.1 Traditional Health Insurance

Fee-for-service, sometimes referred to as indemnity coverage, is a type of insurance plan that provides members with autonomy in choosing physicians and where they receive care, and does not require referrals to specialists (Altman, Cutler, & Zeckhauser, 2000). However, out of pocket expenses are usually higher—including deductibles, which may range from $200-$2,500 (Medical Mutual of Ohio, 2019). Fee-for-service plans were the most common health plans available in the U.S. until managed care plans became more popular.

3.5.2 Managed Care Plans

Managed care plans are currently the most common insurance programs offered in the U.S. These types of plans focus on two aspects of health care: cost and quality. Managed care plans contract with select healthcare providers and organizations to provide services to members at a reduced cost. In addition, these plans focus on preventative health care to improve members' overall health, thus decreasing costs. Other cost-saving incentives include offering generic medications at a reduced price compared to brand. HMOs are one example of a managed care plan. In addition to HMOs, other types of managed care plans include:

- Preferred provider organizations (PPOs): these health plans have a network of physicians, hospitals, and specialists who provide care for members enrolled in the PPO for reduced fees. Unlike an HMO, members do not have to obtain a referral from their primary healthcare provider to see a specialist. Members may choose to see providers who are in or out of network; however, if they select an in-network provider, their cost will be less.

- Point-of-service (POS) plans: a mixture of an HMO and PPO; members are usually required to select a primary healthcare provider and obtain referrals to specialists. Costs will be less if members use an in-network provider.

- High deductible health plans (HDHPs): as the name infers, these plans have higher deductibles than other plans, but the monthly premium is lower. The deductible must be paid by the member before insurance will pay for treatment. Therefore, members of these plans pay less each month in premiums but have higher out-of-pocket expenses when receiving medical care.

HMO Plan

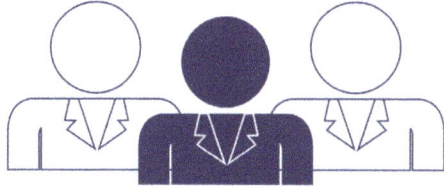

In-network only

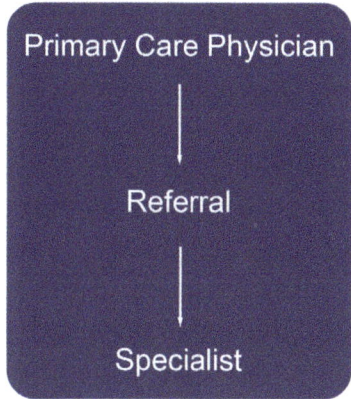

Primary Care Physician
↓
Referral
↓
Specialist

Lower Premium

PPO Plan

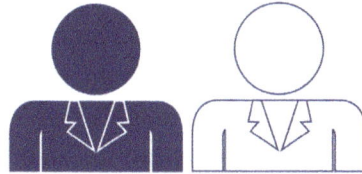

In- or out-of-network

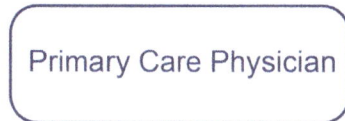

Primary Care Physician

OR

Specialist

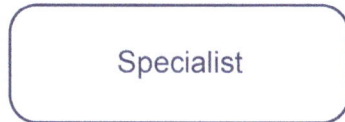

More Flexibility

Figure 3.5: HMO vs. PPO

Source: Original Work
Attribution: Corey Parson
License: CC BY-SA 4.0

Percentage of Covered Workers by Type of Plan

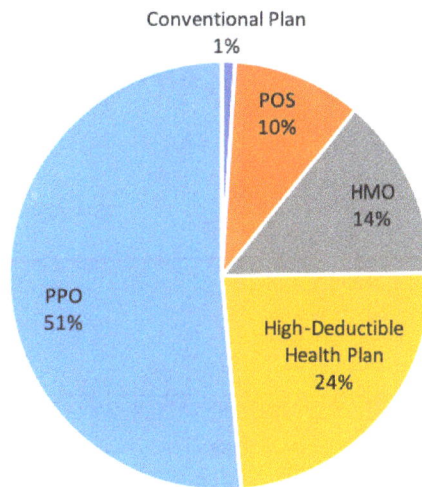

Conventional Plan 1%
POS 10%
HMO 14%
High-Deductible Health Plan 24%
PPO 51%

Figure 3.6: Percentage of Covered Workers by Type of Plan

Source: Kaiser Family Foundation
Attribution: Claxton, Rae, Long, Panchal, & Damico
License: © Kaiser Family Foundation. Used with permission.

3.6 INNOVATIVE NEW APPROACHES TO THE PAYER/PROVIDER MODEL

Traditional (indemnity) plans were the predominant form of insurance until the 1980s when managed care plans were introduced. Traditional plans allowed their members to receive care from any provider and/or healthcare facility with payments based on the care received (fee-for-service). However, this reimbursement structure led to rapid increases in medical costs after providers realized they could increase their revenue by expanding the number of patients healthcare providers treated and ordering more procedures. Health insurance companies countered by increasing patients' cost-shares by raising the amount required for plan deductibles and patient co-payments (Kjesten).

As a result of high insurance costs, many Americans could not afford to purchase health insurance, leading to 44 million uninsured residents by 2013. To combat this issue, President Barack Obama (2008 – 2016) passed a healthcare reform bill, which included the Affordable Care Act (ACA), and the new program began enrollment in fall 2013 (Glied, Ma, Borja, 2017). Included in the ACA, Medicaid coverage was expanded to cover nonelderly adults with incomes below 138 percent of the federal poverty level (FPL) and offered tax credits for individuals with incomes between 100–400% of the FPL. The ACA extended health insurance via a health care marketplace which catered to individuals and small employers and eliminated any pre-existing condition clauses (Garfield, Orgera, Kaiser Family Foundation, & Damico, 2019). The ACA also extended healthcare coverage for children up to age 26 years. As a result, the number of uninsured individuals in the U.S. has fallen from 44 million to 27 million.

Affordable Care Act Coverage Gains Driving Uninsured Rate to Historic Low

Share of population without health insurance

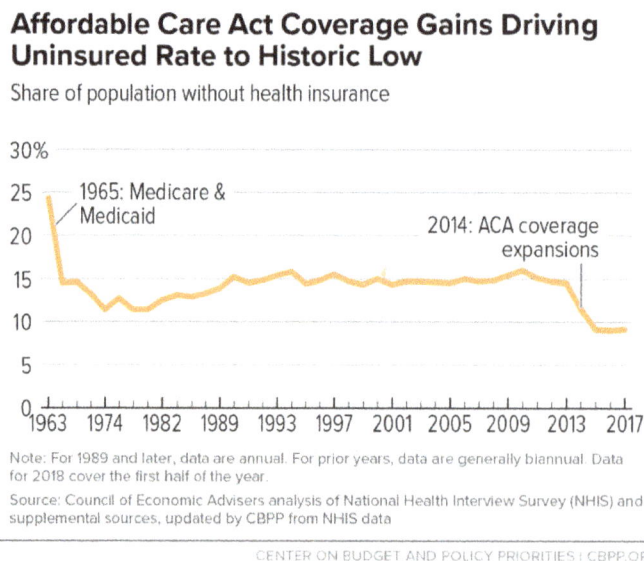

Note: For 1989 and later, data are annual. For prior years, data are generally biannual. Data for 2018 cover the first half of the year.

Source: Council of Economic Advisers analysis of National Health Interview Survey (NHIS) and supplemental sources, updated by CBPP from NHIS data

CENTER ON BUDGET AND POLICY PRIORITIES | CBPP.ORG

Figure 3.7: Affordable Care Act Coverage Gains Driving Uninsured Rate to Historic Low. (This material was created by the Center on Budget and Policy Priorities (www.cbpp.org))

Source: Center on Budget and Policy Priorities

Attribution: Center on Budget and Policy Priorities

License: © Center on Budget and Policy Priorities. Used with permission.

In response to high insurance costs, and in an effort to improve consumer health while controlling costs, insurance companies have developed new, innovative healthcare models that include accountable care organizations (ACOs), Medicare Shared Savings Programs (also referred to as the Patient Centered Medical Home Model, PCMH), and Alternative Quality Contracts (Chernew, Mechanic, Landon, & Safran, 2011; National Committee for Quality Assurance (NCQA), 2019). These models are focused on the *quality* of care beneficiaries receive rather than the *quantity* of services. ACOs include groups of physicians, healthcare organizations, and other providers who work together to provide comprehensive, high-quality care to Medicare patients (Centers for Medicare & Medicaid Services, 2019; ACOs). In exchange for meeting pre-set quality indicators, providers are given financial incentives.

As a result of increased access to health care, as well as medical breakthroughs, Americans are living longer with multiple comorbidities. Due to the complex health needs of an aging population, Medicare recipients often receive care from multiple providers in a variety of settings, and commonly require social and behavioral health care support (Lipson, Rich, Libersky, & Parchman, 2011). The development of the PCMH model addressed these needs by improving beneficiary health through coordinated efforts, enhanced communication between providers and settings, and improved management of chronic health conditions (NCQA, 2019). PCMH models are comprised of five elements:

- Patient-centered orientation toward each patient's unique needs, culture, values, and preferences; support of the patient's self-care efforts; and involvement of the patient in care plans.

- Comprehensive, team-based care that meets the majority of each patient's physical and mental health care needs, including prevention and wellness, acute care, and chronic care which are provided by a cohesive team.

- Care that is coordinated across all elements of a complex healthcare system and connects patients to both medical and social resources in the community.

- Superb access to care that matches patients' needs and preferences, including care provided after hours and alternative methods of communication such as email and telephone.

- A systems-based approach to quality and safety that includes gathering and responding to patient experience data, committing to ongoing quality improvement, and practicing population health management (Lipson, Rich, Libersky, & Parchman, 2011).

For healthcare providers, the benefits of PCMH include improved efficiency and reimbursement support, and lower practice costs (NCQA, 2019).

A third type of healthcare model, alternate quality contracts, addresses the shortcomings of the fee-for-service model by providing healthcare providers with an annual budget for providing care to members, and significant financial incentives for meeting pre-set clinical performance targets (Chernew, Mechanic, Landon, & Safran, 2011). Alternate quality contracts last for a period of five years to provide healthcare providers ample time to meet the clinical targets.

3.7 HEALTH INSURANCE RELATED LAWS AND REGULATIONS

Beginning with the McCarran-Ferguson Act, states were granted the authority to oversee health insurance related products (Kongstvedt, 2020). States have historically regulated issues such as:

- Establishing solvency requirements;
- Requiring coverage for certain medical conditions;
- Establishing requirements for healthcare provider networks;
- Setting standards for medical claim reviews;
- Developing standards for licensing managed care organizations and insurance agents;
- Other consumer protections, such as laws protecting the privacy of health information. (page 232 -233)

However, in 1973 Congress passed the HMO Act which established federal regulatory agency roles and jurisdiction in overseeing managed care policies. Examples of federal laws related to health care include the Affordable Care Act (ACA) and Social Security Act (SSA). Other noteworthy laws include the:

- Employee Retirement Income Security Act of 1974 (ERISA): ERISA was established to set minimum standards for retirement and health plans offered in private industry to provide protection for consumers (U.S. Department of Labor, n.d.). ERISA regulates and sets standards for conduct, reporting and accountability, disclosures, procedural safeguards, and financial and best-interest protection.
- Consolidated Omnibus Budget Reconciliation Act (COBRA) of 1985: COBRA was enacted as an amendment to the ERISA law. This law requires employers with 20 or more employees to offer employees and their families continuing group insurance coverage for limited periods of time during circumstances when coverage would usually end, including:
  - ◇ Voluntary or involuntary job loss;

◇ Reduction in hours worked;

◇ Transition between jobs;

◇ Death, divorce, and other life events (U.S. Department of Labor, n.d.).

Individuals who qualify for COBRA may be required to pay the entire cost of the premium — up to 102 percent of the cost of the plan. If employees cannot afford (or choose not to obtain) COBRA insurance, they may choose to enroll in private health insurance which can be found in the health insurance marketplace.

- Health Insurance Portability and Accountability Act (HIPAA) of 1996: HIPAA is another amendment to ERISA and is most well-known for the protections it offers for personal health information held by covered entities (Heathfield, 2019). This protection extends to patients' and employees' health information. Covered entities include:

  ◇ Health plans (including health insurance companies, HMOs, company health plans) and certain governmental plans such as Medicare and Medicaid;

  ◇ Most health care providers, including most physicians, clinics, hospitals, psychologists, chiropractors, nursing homes, pharmacies, and dentists;

  ◇ Health care clearinghouses – organizations that process health information from other organizations into a standard (i.e., standard electronic format or data content);

  ◇ Business associates—includes individuals or entities who are not employees of the covered entity, including contractors and subcontractors who handle billing practices or process health care claims; companies who administer health plans; lawyers; accountants; IT specialists; and companies that store or destroy medical records (Office for Civil Rights, 2017).

A Covered Entity is one of the following:

A Health Care Provider	A Health Plan	A Health Care Clearinghouse
This includes providers such as: • Doctors • Clinics • Psychologists • Dentists • Chiropractors • Nursing homes • Pharmacies, but only if they transmit any information in an electronic form in connection with a transaction for which HHS has adopted a standard.	This includes: • Health insurance companies • HMOs • Company health plans • Government programs that pay for health care, such as Medicare, Medicaid, and the military and veteran health care programs.	This includes entities that process nonstandard health information they receive from another entity into a standard (i.e., standard electronic format or data content) or vice versa.

Table 3.2

Source: U.S. Department of Health and Human Services
Attribution: U.S. Department of Health and Human Services
License: Public Domain

However, HIPAA also mandates that group plans limit exclusions for preexisting conditions, prohibits discrimination against employees and dependents based on health status, and allows individuals the opportunity to enroll in an individual health insurance plan if a group insurance plan is not available and the individual has exhausted COBRA coverage.

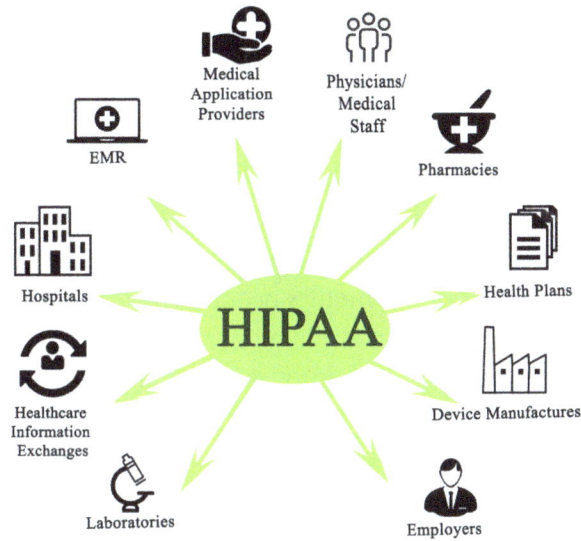

Figure 3.8: Who Must Comply with HIPAA

- Tax Equity and Fiscal Responsibility Act (TEFRA) of 1982: This act allowed states to offer medical assistance to certain children with disabilities who would otherwise not qualify for coverage. Eligibility is not based on parent income and is available to noncitizen children who meet **all** of the following:

  ◇ Under 19 years old;

  ◇ Live with at least one biological or adoptive parent;

  ◇ Certified as disabled;

  ◇ Requires the level of care provided by:

    ▪ A hospital,

    ▪ A nursing home, or

    ▪ An intermediate care facility for persons with mental retardation and related conditions

  ◇ Has an income under 100% of the federal poverty guideline (FPG) for a household size of one (Department of Human Services, 2017).

3.8 OVERSIGHT AND REGULATION OF REIMBURSEMENT PRACTICES

There are two major types of payment practices available: risk-based and non-risk-based. Risk-based payment programs share some portion of financial risk for medical costs with the provider (Kongstvedt, 2020). This method ensures that the financial goals of the provider align with those of the payer and/or employer which helps contain medical costs. In contrast, non-risk-based payment methods do not align the provider's financial goals with the payer and/or employer, but rather reimburses providers a higher payment in correlation with higher costs/ fees. All types of payer practices may choose to participate in non-risk-based payment methods (and most do); however, only HMOs may choose to use risk-based payment methods.

A third type of reimbursement plan is the value-based payment (VBP) program, which bases reimbursement on both costs and quality (or outcomes) and usually involves non-risk-based payment methods that are modified. VBP is less common than other types of reimbursement methods because it is vaguely defined, with some plans focusing mostly on costs OR quality, with no standard definitions or methods in place (Kongstvedt, 2020). One exception is the Medicare fee-for-service (FFS) program.

In an effort to oversee healthcare and reimbursement practices, the federal government has developed regulatory agencies dedicated to this task. In addition, states provide their own agencies to investigate and combat fraud and abuse (Safian, 2009). Listed below are several of the major agencies, along with their roles in health care:

- Centers for Medicare and Medicaid Services (CMS) is an organization within the Department of Health and Human Services (DHHS) that is responsible for regulating Medicare, Medicaid, and the Children's Health Insurance Program (CHIP);

- Comprehensive Error Rate Testing (CERT) was created by CMS to collect data regarding the error rate for claims that were erroneously paid to providers;

- Durable Medical Equipment Regional Carriers (DMERC) regulate and process claims for durable medical equipment (DME) applied for by Medicare beneficiaries;

- Federal Bureau of Investigation (FBI) focuses on investigating both organizations and individuals suspected of defrauding healthcare systems;

- Hospital Payment Monitoring Program (HPMP) is another organization established by CMS to collect data regarding the error rate for Medicare claims erroneously approved by Quality Improvement Organizations (QIOs);

- Joint Commission is an agency that accredits health care organizations that meet quality and safety of care standards; accreditation is one measure used to qualify facilities to participate in programs such as Medicare and Medicaid;

- Medicaid Fraud Control Units (MFCU) are state-run organizations that investigate and prosecute individuals suspected of defrauding

Medicaid, and/or abusing and neglecting patients who receive Medicaid. States receive federal grant money through the Medicare and Medicaid Anti-Fraud and Abuse Amendments of 1997 to operate these agencies.

- Office of Civil Rights (OCR) is an organization within the Department of Health and Human Services that oversees compliance with HIPAA and investigates and prosecutes violations;

- U.S. Department of Justice (DOJ) developed the National Procurement Fraud Task Force to oversee the prevention, detection, and prosecution of procurement fraud (Safian, 2009, pgs. 58-61).

3.9 REGULATORY STATUTES AND PROGRAMS

This section will introduce you to the current laws that are in place to regulate reimbursement practices. It is impossible to include all applicable laws due to the variety of clinical settings in which care is provided. Further, some laws may pertain to certain practice settings but not others. Therefore, only key legislation will be included for review.

- Emergency Medical Treatment and Active Labor Act (EMTALA) was passed in 1986 to ensure that any facility that cares for Medicare patients and provides emergency services will provide medical assessments and/or treatments to stabilize patients in need of emergent care without regard to the patient's ability to pay. Facilities and/or providers found to have violated EMTALA are subject to penalties including termination of the entity's Medicare provider agreement; hospital fines up to $50,000 per violation ($25,000 for hospitals with less than 100 beds); and physician fines of $50,000 per violation. In addition, hospitals may be sued in civil court, and the receiving facility may sue for financial loss related to the other hospital's violation of EMTALA (American College of Emergency Physicians, 2019).

- Federal False Claims Act makes it illegal for anyone to "knowingly submit a false claim to the government or cause another to submit a false claim to the government or knowingly make a false record or statement to get a false claim paid by the government...the reverse false claims section provides liability where one acts improperly – not to get money from the government, but to avoid having to pay money to the government" (DOJ, 2011). According to the FCA, it is not illegal to simply submit a false claim to the government in error; it is illegal to knowingly submit (or cause the submission of) a false claim. Penalties for violating the FCA include fines up to three times the claim amount, plus $11,000 per claim filed. Those individuals found to be in violation are also subject to criminal prosecution and incarceration of up to five years (CMS, Laws, 2015).

- In addition to regulating privacy laws regarding individual and employee health information, HIPAA also mandates the use of diagnostic and procedure codes for reimbursement practices (CMS, 2019). These code sets classify medical diagnoses, procedures, diagnostic tests, treatments, equipment, and supplies.

Code Set	Type of Usage
Current procedural terminology, fourth revision (CPT – 4)	Procedure or type of service by physicians and other providers for inpatient and outpatient care.
Healthcare common procedural coding system (HCPCS)	Codes used by many different types of providers. Level 1 codes and CPT – 4, Level 2 codes are for ambulance, equipment, supplies, and so forth for which there are no CPT – 4 codes.
International classification of diseases, 10th edition, clinical modification (ICD – 10)	Used to report diagnoses in all clinical settings. ICD – 10 replaces Volumes 1 and 2 of ICD – 9 – CM, and ICD – 10 – PCS replaces Volume 3.
National drug codes (NDC)	Used for drugs and biologics.
Code on dental procedures and nomenclature (CDT)	Used for dental procedures and services.

Table 3.3: Standardized Code Sets Mandated by HIPAA

Source: Centers for Medicare and Medicaid Services
Attribution: Centers for Medicare and Medicaid Services
License: Public Domain

Approval for reimbursement, along with the amount of reimbursement, is affected by the code used for billing. Penalties for HIPAA violations range from fines to criminal charges and incarceration up to 10 years. Fines may range from $25,000 per violation category to $1.5 million per violation category.

HIPAA PRIVACY VIOLATION BY TYPES

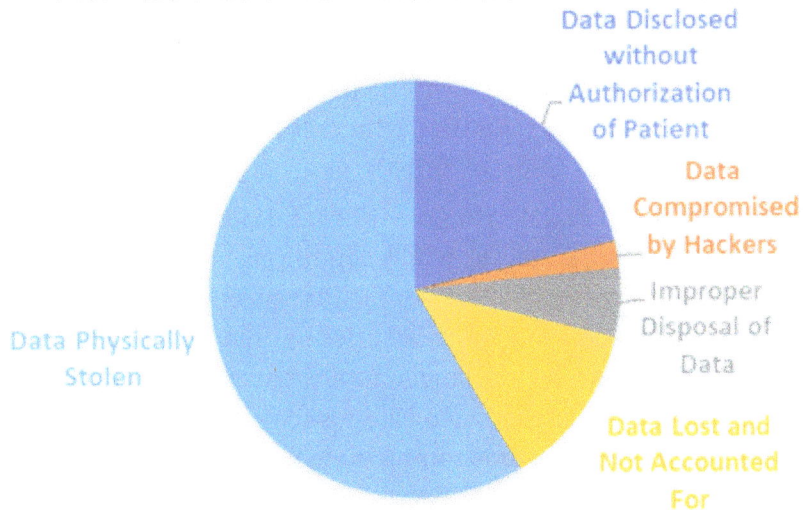

Data Disclosed without Authorization of Patient

Data Compromised by Hackers

Improper Disposal of Data

Data Physically Stolen

Data Lost and Not Accounted For

Figure 3.9: HIPAA Privacy Violation by Types

Source: Original Work
Attribution: Larecia Gill
License: CC BY-SA 4.0

HIPAA Violation Penalties

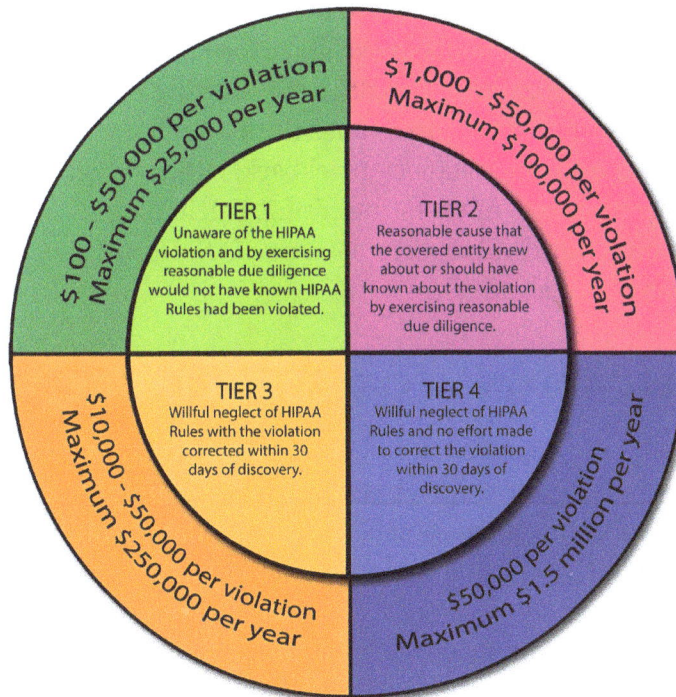

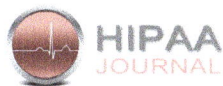

$100 - $50,000 per violation
Maximum $25,000 per year

$1,000 - $50,000 per violation
Maximum $100,000 per year

TIER 1
Unaware of the HIPAA violation and by exercising reasonable due diligence would not have known HIPAA Rules had been violated.

TIER 2
Reasonable cause that the covered entity knew about or should have known about the violation by exercising reasonable due diligence.

TIER 3
Willful neglect of HIPAA Rules with the violation corrected within 30 days of discovery.

TIER 4
Willful neglect of HIPAA Rules and no effort made to correct the violation within 30 days of discovery.

$10,000 - $50,000 per violation
Maximum $250,000 per year

$50,000 per violation
Maximum $1.5 million per year

HIPAA JOURNAL

© HIPAA Journal 2018

Figure 3.10: HIPAA Violation Penalties

Source: HIPAA Journal
Attribution: HIPAA Journal
License: © HIPAA Journal. Used with permission.

- Health Care Fraud and Abuse Control Program (HCFACP) was developed under the auspices of the Office of Inspector General (OIG) and the Department of Justice by HIPAA in an effort to coordinate federal, state, and local law enforcement activities in addressing health care fraud and abuse (U.S. Department of Health and Human Services, Office of Inspector General, 2019).

- The Physician Self-Referral Act – Stark I, II, and III, otherwise known as the Stark Law, specifies conditions under which a provider cannot refer a patient to another facility; specifically, the provider cannot refer patients to other facilities or organizations in which the referring provider has a financial interest/ownership in the facility or organization. This statute also extends to facilities and/or organizations that the referring provider's immediate family has a financial interest in and/or holds ownership (Safian, 2009). Although the Stark Law only regulates referrals for patients who have Medicaid and Medicare, most states also have a version of this law. Penalties for violating the Stark Law may include lifetime exclusion from participating as a Medicare provider, repayment of all Medicare payments received for any referrals that violated the law, and fines.

- Anti-Kickback Law is related to the Stark Law and prohibits a physician from receiving payments in exchange for referring patients to other facilities/organizations. Penalties for violating the anti-kickback law includes fines that are three times the amount of renumeration plus up to $50,000 per instance of kickback. Other penalties may include incarceration and/or exclusion from participating in federal health care programs (Office of Inspector General, U.S. Department of Health & Human Services, 2019).

3.10 IMPLICATIONS FOR COMPLIANCE

In chapter one, the importance of a compliance program was discussed. This chapter expanded on those principles by explaining how compliance with healthcare, and specifically reimbursement practices, are regulated. Multiple agencies are tasked with providing oversight to ensure individuals and organizations comply with the rules and regulations that are in place. As a member of a health care team, all members must practice in a legal and ethical manner and submit to all compliance programs. When members fail to comply, there must be repercussions. The compliance plan, along with the compliance policies and procedures manual, must outline the penalties that will be levied for infractions.

Once a violation has been identified, the first step in the disciplinary action plan includes notifying the individual(s) involved (Safian, 2009). Components of the notification should include:

1. The policy or law that the individual(s) is accused of violating. The notice should be specific enough to allow the accused to understand what they are alleged of violating and keep the focus on only this topic.

2. The evidence and/or information which led to the allegations against the individual. Names of any witnesses or sources should not be shared with the individual to avoid any conflict or prevent harassment.

3. How the investigation will be carried out, what level of disciplinary action may be taken, and who will be involved in the investigative process.

4. Information regarding the individual's right to defend his or her actions, and the right to appeal any disciplinary actions imposed (Safian, 2009).

The level of disciplinary action that should be taken depends on the seriousness of the infraction. Other concerns that should also be considered are whether the accused has a history of prior violations, if they received appropriate training prior to the infraction, and whether the violation was committed intentionally or if it was a mistake. The disciplinary action plan should be progressive and implemented consistently across the organization. The levels of disciplinary action include:

1. Verbal Warning: this level of disciplinary action is reserved for minor infractions such as tardiness. The supervisor usually provides a verbal warning and includes suggested corrective actions that should be taken. The incident should be documented simply by including the time and date of the warning, suggested corrective actions, and the accused individual's response (Safian, 2009).

2. Written Warning: when providing a formal corrective action, the supervisor should use an official disciplinary action form to document the encounter and corrective actions taken (Betterteam, 2019). If additional training is required, the deadline for completing the training should be included in the action plan (Safian, 2009). The accused individual should read the form, provide his or her signature and date, and receive a copy of the signed form.

3. Formal Disciplinary Meeting: this level is reserved for violations that are serious enough to require punitive action such as suspension (with or without pay), demotion, and/or exclusion from a company benefit such as an annual bonus (Safian, 2009). The meeting should be documented using an official disciplinary action form, signed by the supervisor and accused, and a copy given to the individual.

4. Termination: this level is the highest with the most severe consequence and is reserved for serious infractions including major violations, or for individuals who continue to violate policy despite being warned repeatedly (Safian, 2009). Due to the seriousness of the violation and

disciplinary action, the supervisor must provide thorough documentation of all elements previously mentioned, along with copies of previous warnings or notifications given to the individual, and all other records that influenced the decision to terminate.

3.11 SUMMARY

Historically, insurance plans have not been available or affordable for many Americans. As the types of plans available have evolved, so too has the focus from a fee-for-service to a quality (outcome) metric. Americans now have more options for insurance plans than ever before, yet still struggle with affordability. In an effort to provide affordable options, new innovative insurance plans are being developed. As a consumer, it is vital to remain current on such changes to make educated decisions regarding your insurance coverage.

In order to protect citizens from fraud, abuse, and/or loss of personal health information, governmental organizations provide oversite and governance of the insurance industry. Health compliance programs are one way employers ensure they remain current with policies and legislation regarding insurance regulations. Failure to comply with compliance programs may result in disciplinary actions up to and including termination. Therefore, it is crucial that all members of the health care team are aware of the regulations and laws and adhere to policies and procedures. Ignorance of the law is not a defense and may result in punitive measures from the employer, as well as the governing organization.

3.12 DISCUSSION QUESTIONS

1. Discuss two examples of innovative insurance plans and how they attempt to contain health care costs.

2. Compare and contrast the types of insurance.

3. Find a recent case in the media regarding a HIPPA violation. Discuss issues regarding the case including what action violated HIPPA, what punishment was imposed, and what was the maximum penalty that could be imposed.

4. Describe the various penalties that may be imposed for noncompliance with reimbursement practices.

3.13 KEY TERM DEFINITIONS

1. Accountable Care Organizations (ACOs) – a healthcare organization that ties provider reimbursement to quality metrics and reductions in the cost of care.

2. Electronic Health Record (EHR) – an electronic version of a patient's

medical history; may include all of the key administrative clinical data relevant to the patient's care including demographics, progress notes, problems, medications, vital signs, past medical history, immunizations, and laboratory and radiologic reports.

3. Federal Poverty Level (FPL) – a measure of income used by the U.S. government to determine who is eligible for subsidies, programs, and benefits.

4. Fee-for-service (FFS) – a payment model where services are unbundled and paid for separately; payment is dependent on the quantity of care rather than quality of care.

5. Health Maintenance Organization (HMO) – one type of insurance plan that includes a set of network providers, hospitals, and other healthcare providers who have agreed to accept payment at a certain level for any services they provide.

6. Preferred Provider Organizations (PPO) – a type of insurance plan that provides maximum benefits if members use an in-network provider, but still provides some coverage for out-of-network providers.

7. Primary Care Physician (PCP) – sometimes referred to as a primary care provider, a PCP is a healthcare professional who is chosen by or assigned to a patient, provides primary health care, and acts as a gatekeeper to control access to other medical providers and/or services.

3.14 REFERENCES:

Agency for Healthcare Research and Quality, AHRQ. (2011, October). Ensuring that Patient-Centered Medical Homes effectively serve patient with complex health needs. Patient-Centered Medical Home Decisionmaker Brief.

Altman, D., Cutler, D., & Zeckhauser, R. (2000) Enrollee mix, treatment intensity, and cost in competing indemnity and HMO plans. National Bureau of Economic Research Working Paper 7832. *Journal of Health Economics, 22*(1), 23-45.

American College of Emergency Physicians. (2019) *EMTALA Fact Sheet.* Retrieved from https://www.acep.org/life-as-a-physician/ethics--legal/emtala/emtala-fact-sheet/#:~:targetText=The%20Emergency%20Medical%20Treatment%20and,has%20remained%20an%20unfunded%20mandate

Betterteam. (2019, July 29). Disciplinary Action. Retrieved from https://www.betterteam.com/disciplinary-action

Center on Budget and Policy Priorities. (2019). *Chart Book: Accomplishments of Affordable Care Act.* Washington, DC.: Center on Budget and Policy Priorities.

Centers for Medicare & Medicaid Services, CMS. (2019). Accountable Care Organizations (ACOs). Retrieved from CMS.gov

Centers for Medicare & Medicaid Services, CMS. (2019). Code Sets Overview.

Retrieved from https://www.cms.gov/Regulations-and-Guidance/Administrative-Simplification/Code-Sets/index.html

Centers for Medicare & Medicaid Services, CMS. (2015). Laws against health care fraud resource guide. Retrieved from https://www.cms.gov/Medicare-Medicaid-Coordination/Fraud-Prevention/Medicaid-Integrity-Education/Downloads/fwa-laws-resourceguide.pdf

Centers for Medicare & Medicaid Services, CMS. (2019). Medicaid eligibility. Retrieved from https://www.medicaid.gov/medicaid/eligibility/index.html

Chernew, M.E., Mechanic, R.E., Landon, B.E., & Safran, D.G. (2011). Private-payer innovation in Massachusetts: The 'Alternative Quality Contract'. *Health Affairs, 30*(1), 51-61. DOI: 10.1377/hlthaff.2010.0980

Cystic Fibrosis Foundation. (n.d.) The Insurance Basics retrieved from https://www.cff.org/Assistance-Services/How-Compass-Helps-People-With-CF-and-Their-Families/Understanding-Insurance/Your-Insurance-Plan/The-Insurance-Basics/

Claxton, G., Rae, M., Long, M., Panchal, N., & Damico, A. (2015*) Kaiser Family Foundation Employer Health Benefits: 2015 Annual Survey.* Menlo Park, CA.: Henry J. Kaiser Family Foundation

Department of Human Services. (2017). Medical Assistance for children with disabilities – TEFRA option. Retrieved from https://mn.gov/dhs/people-we-serve/people-with-disabilities/health-care/health-care-programs/programs-and-services/ma-tefra.jsp

Department of Justice, DOJ. (2011). The False Claims Act: A Primer. Retrieved from https://www.justice.gov/sites/default/files/civil/legacy/2011/04/22/C-FRAUDS_FCA_Primer.pdf

Employee Disciplinary Action Form. (n.d.). Retrieved from https://www.centenary.edu

Garfield, R., Orgera, K., Kaiser Family Foundation, & Damico, A. (2019). *The uninsured and the ACA: A Primer – Key facts about health insurance and the uninsured amidst changes to the Affordable Care Act.* Menlo Park, CA.: Henry J. Kaiser Family Foundation.

Glied, S.A., Ma, S., Borja, A. (2017). Effects of the Affordable Care Act on health care access. The Commonwealth Fund retrieved from https://www.commonwealthfund.org/publications/issue-briefs/2017/may/effect-affordable-care-act-health-care-access

Heathfield, S.M. (2019). Health Insurance Portability and Accountability Act. The balance careers: Human Resources, Compensation. Retrieved from https://www.thebalancecareers.com/health-insurance-portability-and-accountability-act-1918152

HHS.gov. (2017). Health Information Privacy: Covered entities & business associates. Retrieved from https://www.hhs.gov/hipaa/for-professionals/covered-entities/index.html

HIPAA Journal. (2018). What is a HIPAA violation? Retrieved https://www.hipaajournal.com/what-is-a-hipaa-violation/#:~:targetText=What%20are%20the%20

Penalties%20for,per%20violation%20category%2C%20per%20year

Kaiser Family Foundation. (2019). *Where are states today? Medicaid and CHIP eligibility levels for children, pregnant women, and adults.* Kaiser Family Foundation. Retrieved from https://www.kff.org/medicaid/fact-sheet/where-are-states-today-medicaid-and-chip/

Klees, B.S., Wolfe, C.J., & Curtis, C.A. (2009). *Medicare & Medicaid: Title XVIII and Title XIX of the Social Security Act.* Centers for Medicare & Medicaid Services, Department of Health and Human Services.

Kongstvedt, P. (2020). *Health insurance and managed care: What they are and how they work (5th Ed).* Burlington, MA: Jones & Bartlett Learning, LLC.

Lipson D, Rich E, Libersky J, Parchman M. (2011, October). *Ensuring That Patient-Centered Medical Homes Effectively Serve Patients With Complex Health Needs.* (Prepared by Mathematica Policy Research under Contract No. HHSA290200900019I TO 2.) AHRQ Publication No. 11-. Rockville, MD: Agency for Healthcare Research and Quality.

Medical Mutual of Ohio. (2019). HMO vs. PPO insurance plan. Retrieved from https://www.medmutual.com/For-Individuals-and-Families/Health-Insurance-Education/Compare-Health-Insurance-Plans/HMO-vs-PPO-Insurance.aspx

National Committee for Quality Assurance, NCQA. (2019). PCMH benefits to practices, clinicians and patients. Retrieved from https://www.ncqa.org/programs/health-care-providers-practices/patient-centered-medical-home-pcmh/benefits-support/benefits/

Office for Civil Rights. (2019). U.S. Department of Health & Human Services. Health Information Privacy: Your rights under HIPAA. Retrieved from https://www.hhs.gov/hipaa/for-individuals/guidance-materials-for-consumers/index.html

Office of Inspector General, U.S. Department of Health & Human Services. (2019). *A roadmap for new physicians: Fraud & abuse laws.* Retrieved from https://oig.hhs.gov/compliance/physician-education/01laws.asp

Quora. (2018). What is HIPAA compliance? Retrieved from https://www.quora.com/What-is-HIPAA-Compliance-1

Safian, S.C. (2009). *Essentials of Health Care Compliance.* Clifton Park, NY: Delmar, Cengage Learning.

Social Security Administration. (2019). *Medicare premiums: Rules for higher-income beneficiaries.* Retrieved from https://www.ssa.gov/pubs/EN-05-10536.pdf

Sunshine, P. (2016, June). How does an HMO plan work? 3 Tips for switching to an HMO plan. *Health Insurance.* Retrieved October 24, 2019 from https://insights.ibx.com/how-does-an-hmo-plan-work-3-tips-for-switching-from-a-ppo-to-an-hmo-plan/

U.S. Department of Health and Human Services, Office of Inspector General. (2019). *Health Care Fraud and Abuse Control Program Report.* Retrieved from https://oig.hhs.gov/reports-and-publications/hcfac/index.asp

U.S. Department of Labor, USDOL. (n.d.). *Health Plans & Benefits: Continuation of Health Coverage – COBRA*. Retrieved from https://www.dol.gov/general/topic/health-plans/cobra

U.S. Department of Labor, USDOL. (n.d.). *Health Plans & Benefits: ERISA*. Retrieved from https://www.dol.gov/general/topic/health-plans/erisa

Wolf, L. (2019). What does ERISA cover? The balance careers: Women in business, Basics. Retrieved from https://www.thebalancecareers.com/what-is-erisa-law-3515060

4 Quality Improvement

4.1 LEARNING OBJECTIVES

1. Identify the essential components that organizations need for quality improvement and patient safety.
2. Discuss the future of tailored therapeutics.
3. Analyze the issues surrounding producers of medical products.

4.2 INTRODUCTION

Quality improvement and patient safety in healthcare are the most important aspects when caring for patients. This chapter will focus on the fundamentals of patient safety and quality improvement for healthcare professionals to improve the health of patients, families, and communities while lowering costs. This chapter will also provide knowledge of various topics related to quality improvement as it relates to healthcare compliance.

4.3 KEY TERMS

- Quality Improvement
- Risk Management
- Evidence-based practice
- Patient-centered care
- Workflow Design

The Institute of Medicine defines quality of care as the degree to which health services for individuals and populations increase the likelihood of desired health outcomes and are consistent with current professional knowledge (Institute of Medicine, 2001). Quality improvements in healthcare are vital to improve patient safety while reducing costs. In 2001, the Institute of Medicine's *Crossing the*

Quality Chasm: A New Health System for the 21st Century provided a guide for changes that must take place in U.S. hospitals and healthcare organizations to ensure the delivery of quality of care. The alarming statistic that approximately 98,000 hospital patients died in 1999 due to preventable medical errors highlighted the need for this guide (Institute of Medicine, 2001). Also, a study out of Johns Hopkins University states that medical errors are the third-leading cause of death in the U.S. (Johns Hopkins Medicine, 2016).

The guide from this report listed six components of *quality* healthcare: safety, effectiveness, efficiency, equity, timeliness, and patient-centeredness (Whedon, 2016). In order to move forward with discussing quality, we will first define these components.

Patient safety is vital in healthcare. Safe and effective care is secure for patients and utilizes cutting edge healthcare science to serve as the standard in care delivery. Healthcare technologies are designed to improve patient safety and streamline workflow while improving patient care quality (McGonigle & Mastrian, 2018). Healthcare providers must evaluate errors carefully and change processes and protocols so that future errors do not occur. Due to the rapid changes in technology, error reporting should prompt continuous quality improvements within the healthcare system.

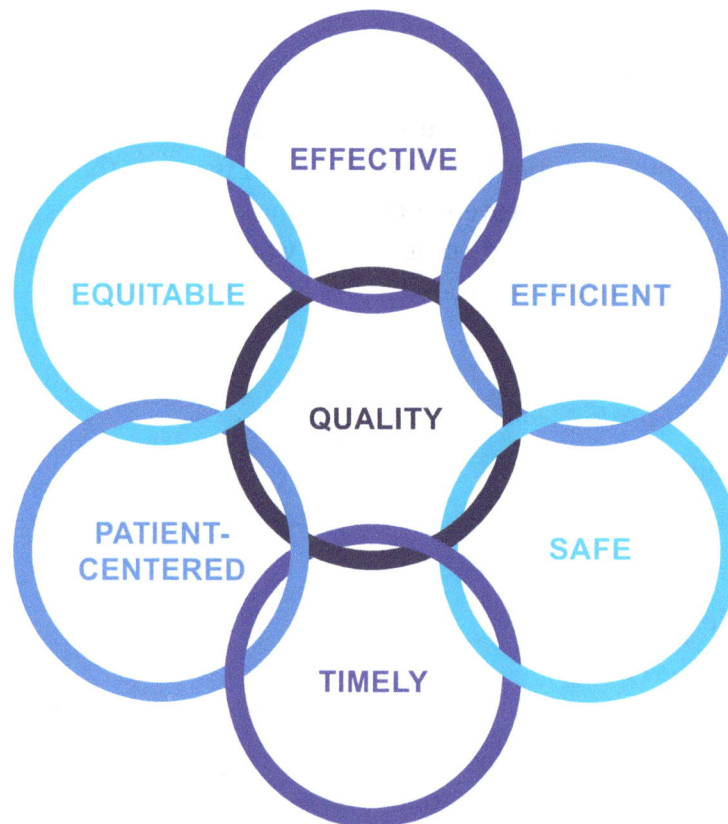

Figure 4.1: Components of Quality Healthcare

Source: Original Work
Attribution: Corey Parson
License: CC BY-SA 4.0

Think About This Scenario

A patient arrives at the emergency room department complaining of difficulty breathing. The doctor comes into the room to examine the patient and orders IV heparin (a blood thinner) because the doctor believes the patient may have a pulmonary embolism. The nurse administers the heparin on a misprogrammed IV pump, causing the patient to hemorrhage and die. The pump is designed to alarm using the dose checking technology; however, the nurse decided to bypass this feature.

Here is another scenario: A nurse is administering medication to a patient and goes to the OMNICELL (medication dispensing equipment) to gather the medication. The system alerts the nurse that she is getting the incorrect medication; however, the nurse bypasses the alerts several times and continues to retrieve the medication assuming that the pharmacy had placed it in the wrong location when the OMNICELL was filled. The nurse failed to realize she was looking at what she thought was a generic name for the medication, when she was actually pulling an entirely different medication and the system was attempting to stop the nurse from making a huge mistake. The nurse moved forward with administering the incorrect medication to the patient, and the patient dies.

Technology and electronic equipment can be great for healthcare, but if not used properly they can cause great harm to the patient. Healthcare professionals, therefore, must always keep the safety of the patient as a top priority when using various medical technology. Busy healthcare professionals rely heavily on equipment with the assumption that doing so will improve outcomes for the patient. Healthcare professionals must always be alert and triple check, though, before administering medications or performing any tasks that can potentially cause the patient harm. Technology is not always the answer with regards to patient safety.

In order to be efficient, the care should also be cost effective without much waste. Many hospitals are using the lean management system in order to reduce costs while caring for patients. Between 2001 and 2003, hospital infection rates alone accounted for over 9,000 deaths and $2.6 billion in excess costs (Hoeft & Pryor, 2016). This issue prompted standardizing nursing processes to improve direct patient care, communication, and medication administration (Boettcher, Hunter, McGonagle, 2019). Workflow designs are important to help facilitate patient care quality while reducing wastes and costs. If a healthcare provider has to go out of the patient's room every time they need to document vital information into the chart, then the patient is placed at risk without their having the most up to date information documented. For example, if a patient is on pain medication directly after surgery while in the hospital, and the nurse comes into the patient's room to administer the medication but is distracted by doing other things for the patient and then leaves the room failing to document the "as needed" medication into the chart, this oversight places the patient at risk for being given a duplicate dose by another nurse. Having computer stations in every hospital room helps to eliminate this problem and allows the nurse the opportunity to document vital information in a timely manner while also reducing costs, eliminating waste, and reducing potential harm to the patient.

4.4 PATIENT-CENTERED CARE

The adoption of patient and family centered care is increasing within healthcare organizations across the U.S. to facilitate engagement of patients and families as partners in their care (DeRosa, Nelso, Delgado, 2019). In the past, healthcare was driven by the fee-for-service model. The insurance and federal payers reimbursed the providers and healthcare facilities based on the service that was provided. Currently, payment models are moving away from the fee-for-service model and are moving instead toward reimbursements for prevention and value-based care, also termed pay for performance. New quality models for payments are emerging to include the Patient Centered Medical Home model and Accountable Care Organizations (Accountable Care Organization, 2015). Providers are held as being accountable for the quality of care the patient receives.

Due to the different interpretations of what quality means, standardized measurements were developed and established to offer healthcare providers a guide to use; they are listed as Healthcare Effectiveness Data and Information Set (HEDIS measures). These measurements are also used for more than 90% of the health plans in the U.S. (Whedon, 2016). HEDIS provide a set of standardized performance measures for healthcare performance-reporting to hold organizations accountable for achieving results. The focus is on prevention and screening, access to and satisfaction with various health care services, and measures that are used for specific procedures. The purpose of HEDIS measures is to prevent healthcare quality's failing to rise in proportion to rising healthcare costs. Therefore, HEDIS can encourage accountability and quality in healthcare.

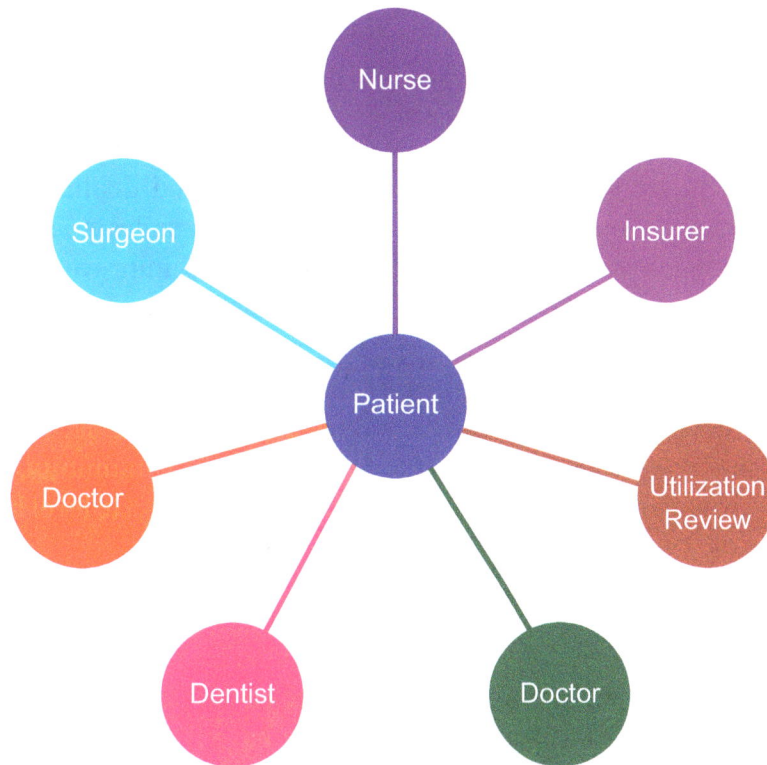

Figure 4.2: Patient Centered Medical Home Model

Example

Here's an example of this new quality payment model in this scenario: A 55 year old female patient with a diagnosis of hypertension and diabetes visits the primary care physician for a routine yearly visit. The provider views the quality metrics that are populating in the electronic medical record based upon this patient's age, gender, and diagnoses listed in the chart. The provider therefore orders a mammogram, blood work, and a referral to podiatry. The provider is now accountable for ensuring results return from the blood work, mammogram, and a physician note from podiatry. The patient must now be notified for any follow up visits or changes to medication if they are needed. This shows the provider is using the HEDIS measures that are populated in all electronic medical records and that reports can now be used based upon if the provider "met" these quality measures.

The importance of patient-centered care focuses on not only the patient's diagnosis but also the patient's health and well-being. Patient Centered Medical Home models encourage the providers to improve quality of patient care. Not all medical clinics have the status of "Patient Centered Medical Home," but many are striving to move in this direction. Many clinics strive to attain a Patient Centered Medical Home status. In order for a clinic to be recognized with this status, the clinic must meet a minimum of six structural standards, including the following: patient-centered access, team-based care, population health management, care management, care coordination and transitions, and quality performance and improvements. Population health management includes treating patients with similar diagnoses using these quality guidelines to improve a community. For example, many ambulatory clinics are integrated into a population health management database where certain quality metrics are monitored over time to view the outcomes of a large population of patients. One example of a quality metric used in the population health management database is using diabetic patients to answer such questions as the following: In a community, how many diabetic patients are monitored and maintain a Hemoglobin A1c level below 7%?

4.5 CARE COORDINATION

Care coordination is vital to patient-centered medical care. Oftentimes, payers such as insurance companies hire medical staff to call patients and make sure the patients are taking their medication, the patients have the right medication, and the patients are being followed by the primary care physician. Care coordination helps to improve quality care as well as reduce the number of hospitalizations. Transition of care is where medical staff offers additional support and often sees the patient during the "in between time" after discharge from an inpatient hospital stay and before the patient's office visit with a primary care physician. This supports the patient by ensuring they understand the medication regime and by monitoring the patients for any adverse symptoms or problems before they see their physician, all of which assists in reducing the amount of emergency room visits and hospitalizations.

4.6 EVIDENCE-BASED PRACTICE

Evidence-based practice is defined as the conscientious use of current best evidence to make decisions about patient care (Melnyk, 2015). Healthcare professionals are in the driver's seat for improving healthcare quality while reducing costs. It takes the employees who actually perform the daily tasks of caring for patients to be able to see the results and also to give suggestions for better ways in providing care or performing certain tasks.

Example

Imagine going into the hospital and having a procedure that required anesthesia and a Foley catheter to be placed to capture urine for a short period of time. The Foley catheter is a collection bag with a tube inserted into the patient's bladder to collect urine. After surgery, the nurse fails to empty the bag routinely, does not offer assistance in hygiene, and hangs the bag above the level of the bladder. All of these choices are extremely bad for the patient and provide a breeding ground for infection. Now, antibiotics must be initiated to help cure the patient's infection, and the catheter must be removed. Evidence-based practice has shown best practices for staff when caring for patients with Foley catheters. New evidence indicates to eliminate all use of Foley catheters in healthcare settings if at all possible. New medical product inventions are becoming available for healthcare workers to use in place of Foley catheters. This development occurred because of evidence-based practice in healthcare, which is used to guide clinical practice interventions, and due to the efforts of curious and inquisitive clinicians who are constantly working to improve patient care. Healthcare workers can have a positive impact on future changes of processes, protocols, and technology to improve the quality of patient care.

4.7 QUALITY CONTROL & WORKFLOW DESIGN

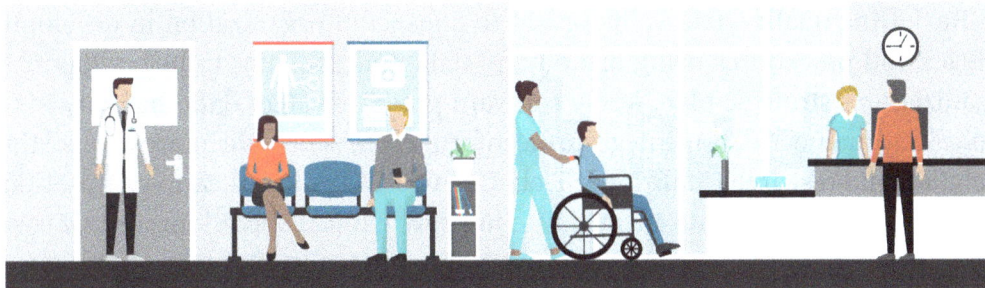

Figure 4.3: Healthcare Workflow Design

Source: 123rf.com
Attribution: User "elenabsl"
License: elenabsl © 123rf.com. Used with permission.

Workflow design is where healthcare professionals can map out processes within a healthcare organization to identify where improvements or changes need to be made (McBride & Tietze, 2019). The goal of workflow design is to improve the quality of patient care, reduce patient wait times, and improve patient safety.

Think About This Scenario

A physician in an internal medicine office sends a patient's prescription electronically to the pharmacy. The medication was an antibiotic to help cure an upper respiratory infection. The physician tells the patient that they can pick up their prescription from their pharmacy after they leave the clinic. However, after the physician enters the medication into the electronic e-prescribing system and signs the order, the physician changes their mind and decides that a different antibiotic would be better for the patient. The patient presents to the pharmacy and picks up two different antibiotics to take. The pharmacist did not call and question the order but instead filled both prescriptions for the patient. The patient presents back to the physician's office the next day with severe abdominal discomfort. This is where workflow design and quality of care can come together. How could have this situation been handled differently? The physician could have simply asked the nurse to phone the pharmacy to let them know of the changes that were made for the patient prior to the patient leaving. Not doing this caused undue harm to the patient and could have potentially caused severe harm had another medication been prescribed. Workflow designs should be built into discussions when related to compliance, quality, and patient safety.

4.8 DATA ANALYSIS AND ANALYTICS

Reviewing quality data is important to engage an organization in developing policies and procedures using meaningful data and analytics to help support an organization's strategic plan. Many software programs align data that consists of clinical and financial data to integrate the information, which can improve reporting, analytics, and research (McBride & Tietze, 2019). Many healthcare organizations, though, struggle to use data effectively to improve clinical operations, reduce costs, and improve research. According to the National Quality Strategy (NQS, 2019), data analysis and analytics have three areas to focus on: better care, healthy people and communities, and affordable care. Data must be entered into systems correctly for the data to be used meaningfully. Charts, bars, graphs, and flowsheets can be used to showcase data that is essential for quality reporting purposes, payments, research improvements in workflow designs, and enhancements to policies and procedures.

4.9 QUALITY REPORTING

The success of the National Quality Strategy depends upon the ability of providers and staff to successfully utilize data to improve quality metrics and increase patient satisfaction scores (Sewell, 2019). Quality metrics in healthcare are vital to improve patient care, foster a healthier community, and lower healthcare costs. Measurement is the first step for improvement. Patient satisfaction surveys are one technique many healthcare organizations utilize to make improvements in patient care. These surveys are often sent to the patient after a hospital stay, and organizations will often call patients to complete a survey via phone as well. Around 2008, the Centers for Medicaid and Medicare set requirements for hospitals to survey patients regarding their experiences from their stay (CMS.gov, 2012). A tool, called the Health Consumer Assessment of Health Providers and Systems (HCAPS), was developed as a standardized survey tool designed for discharged patients' experiences. The data collected from these surveys must be reported to the Centers for Medicaid and Medicare, where they are tracked over time and benchmarked to other hospitals. This data is also available for the public to view. If hospitals choose to not participate in these surveys, then they will receive a financial reduction in payment from federal payers for their patients' hospital stays.

The quality of nursing care can influence a hospital's performance in some of the most core areas within the HCAHPS. For more specific data, some nurse leaders in organizations choose to participate in a survey called the National Database of Nursing Quality Indicators (NDNQI) (Sewell, 2019). This is a survey specific to the nursing care a patient receives during their hospital stay. Hospitals usually will submit nursing data to this national database; the data is then analyzed and reports are given back to the hospital. Nurse leaders and nurse managers can then synthesize the data related to their specific units to focus on the goal of improving the quality of patient care. Some examples of this data include nurse to patient ratios, falls, nursing turnovers, pressure ulcers, infections, restraint use, and nosocomial infections (Press Ganey, 2018). For example, if a patient comes in to stay at the hospital after a recent ortho surgery and then develops a pressure ulcer or experiences a fall with injury, these costs are not covered by federal payers and will often lead to longer patient stays in which the hospital will have to take ownership of the costs related to these events. These events not only have a negative impact on the hospital financially, but also influence their scores from the surveys, which can cause them to experience a larger negative impact. It is therefore imperative that hospitals have surveys and monitor their data and results to improve patient care while lowering costs.

4.10 IMPLICATIONS FOR COMPLIANCE & SUMMARY

How does quality affect compliance in healthcare? Many healthcare organizations have compliance departments that view and monitor tasks, protocols, and other activities to ensure patient care is not jeopardized when it comes to quality care. Compliance is an important factor to monitor because it ensures that tasks are being performed in a timely manner, results are reviewed efficiently, and standards of practice are being followed. Oftentimes, risk management departments must get involved with issues that concern patient safety, or situations that arise and cause harm, even death, to patients. Risk management is a department in which a hospital employs several nurses and medical lawyer(s) whose roles are to investigate events that impact patient safety, patient harm, and death related events. Their roles are vital to the hospital and help improve quality, prevent errors from occurring by setting appropriate policies and procedures in place, and educate staff on the required protocols.

Think About This Scenario

A patient goes into the operating room to have a scheduled knee surgery. The patient was going to have his right knee operated on and a knee replacement performed. However, the surgeon operates on the left knee instead. The patient did not consent for his left knee to be operated on. The consent was for the right knee. Now the patient has endured a long surgery that he must heal from on the wrong lower extremity. The risk management department gets involved in case there is litigation that comes from this situation. Also, the compliance department needs to be involved to audit what went wrong. Did the physician fail to mark the wrong leg? Did the nurse fail to check behind the physician to ensure the correct leg was being operated on? Was the "time-out" procedure not followed? How do things like this example go wrong in health care? Sadly, the patient had to go back into the operating room to have another surgery. The hospital will have to endure the costs of the first surgery and hope for litigation not to occur. Compliance gets involved to set standards of care and policies and procedures so that scenarios like this example do not recur. Staff must be trained on any new policies and procedures as well. Adherence to these new policies and procedures must occur in an effort to prevent harm to patients.

Healthcare organizations must go through accreditation processes that are designed to require the organization to self-evaluate and report, maintain compliance regulations, and be transparent with information (Barata, Cunha, Santos, 2018). The shift in payment models already discussed in this chapter also has significant compliance implications. Quality patient care and value-based care are now linked and tied to payments to providers and healthcare organizations, as compared to previous payment models in which quality was not the focus. Compliance departments should connect with various departments within the clinical setting in an organization, especially on matters related to preventing infections and ensuring patient safety. Oftentimes, healthcare organizations operate in "silos" where staff and departments do not communicate with each other and the complete big picture can often be missed. In previous years, healthcare compliance departments were more focused on billing, physician agreements with payer sources, and laws and regulations. Now, compliance should focus on patient care and must extend to the clinical and quality areas within a healthcare organization (Smith, Welker, & Zeko, 2019). Due to rapid changes in healthcare, especially related to quality, payments can now be affected and penalties and incentives can be given. This topic will be discussed further in the technology chapter. "Hospitals must bring the bedside and the business side together to communicate and collaborate on compliance" to allow risks to be managed in a way to improve the lives of patients and make a positive impact on the organization's financial growth (Smith, Welker, Zeko, 2019).

4.11 DISCUSSION QUESTIONS:

1. What is the difference in the compliance department and the risk management department in a healthcare setting? What are the roles and functions of each? Explain.

2. What is the difference between fee-for-service and pay-for-performance? Why are insurance payers and federal payers concerned with quality as it relates to reimbursement?

3. Should providers continue to be paid by a healthcare organization if their quality scores are poor? Why or why not?

4. What are your thoughts on rating a provider based on quality care? (Much like rating a restaurant or a hotel where it is visible and published on the internet)

5. How can population health improve quality of care?

4.12 KEY TERM DEFINITIONS

1. Quality Improvement—a framework which is used to improve how care is delivered to patients.

2. Risk Management—any activity, process, or policy to reduce liability for a patient's safety and financial wellbeing.

3. Evidence-based practice—the use of current best evidence in making decisions about patient care.

4. Patient-centered care—providing care that is respectful and responsive to individual patient preferences, needs, and values and ensure that these choices guide all clinical decisions.

5. Workflow Design—the flow of work through time and space to encompass all activities, technologies, and people to promote and provide quality healthcare.

4.13 REFERENCES

Accountable Care Organization 2015 Program Analysis Quality Performance Standards Narrative Measures Specifications. (2019, October 3). Retrieved from The Centers for Medicare and Medicaid Services, 2015: www.cms.gov/Medicare/Medicare-Fee-for-service-payment/sharedsavingsprogram/downloads/ACO-NarrativeMeasures-Specs.pdf

Ahmad, F., Norman, C., O'Campo, P. (2012). What is needed to implement a Computer-Assisted Health Risk Assessment Tool? An Exploratory Concept Mapping Study. *BMC Med Inform, 12*(1), pg. 149.

American Recovery & Reinvestment Act of 2009. Retrieved from: http://www. govtractus/congress/billepd?bill=h111-1.

Barata, J., Cunha, P., & Santos, A. (2018). Mind the Gap: Assessing Alignment between Hospital Quality and its Information Systems. *Information Technology for Development, 24* (2), pg. 315-332.

Berner, E. (2009). Clinical Decision Support Systems: State of the Art. Retrieved from: http://healthit.ahrq.gov/sites/default/files/docs/page/pdf.

Boettcher, P., Hunter, R., & McGonagle, P. (2019). Using Lean Principles of Standard Work to Improve Clinical Nursing Performance. *Nursing Economics Volume 37 Number 3*, 152-163.

Campbell, R. (2013). The Five Rights of Clinical Decision Support: CDS Tools Helpful for Meeting Meaningful Use. *Journal of AHIMA. 84*(10), pg. 42-47.

CMS.gov. (2012). *Stage 2 Overview tipsheet.* Retrieved from https://www.cms.gov/ Regulations-and-Guidance/Legislation/EHRIncentivePrograms/Downlaods/ Stage2Overview_Tipsheet.pdf

DeRosa, A.,Nelson, B., Delgado, D. & Mages, K.; *Journal of the Medical Library Association,* July2019; 107(3): p.314-322.

Greenes, R. (2014). *Clinical decision support: The road to broad adoption* (2nd ed.). Philadelphia, PA: Elsevier.

Hoeft, S. &. (2016). *The power of ideas to transform healthcare: Engaging staff by building daily lean management systems.* Boca Raton, FL: CRC Press, Taylor & Francis Group.

Institute of Medicine. (2001). *Crossing the Quality Chasm: A New Health System for the 21st Century.* Washington, D.C.: National Academies Press.

Joshi,M., Ranson, E., Nash, D. & Ranson, S.(2014). *The healthcare quality book. Vision, Strategy, and Tools (3rd ed).* Chicago, IL: Health Administration Press Marketing

Kiron, D., Ferguson, R., & Prentice, P. (2013). *From value to vision: Reimaging the possible with data analytics: What makes companies that are great at analytics different from everyone else.* (Research Report). Cambridge, MA: MIT Sloan Management Review. Retrieved from: http://www.sas.com/content/dam/SAS/ en_us/doc/whitepaper2/reimagining-possible-data-analytics-106272.pdf

Melnyk, B. &.-O. (2015). Evidence-based practice in nursing & healthcare. A guide to best practice. In B. &.-O. Melnyk, *Evidence-based practice in nursing & healthcare. A guide to best practice (3rd ed.)* (pp. 3-23). Philadelphia, PA: Wolters Kluwer.

McBride, S. & Tietze, M. (2019). *Nursing informatics for the advanced practice nurse (2nd ed).* New York, NY: Springer Publishing Company (Accountable Care Organization 2015 Program Analysis Quality Performance Standards Narrative Measures Specifications, 2019)

McGonigle, D. & Mastrian, K. (2018). *Nursing Informatics and the foundation of knowlede (4thed)*. Burlington, MA: Jones & Bartlett Learning

National Quality Stategy. Healthcare Research and Quality. (March 2017). Retrieved from: https://www.ahrq.gov/workingforquality/about/index.html.

Press Ganey. (2018). Nursing quality (NDNQI). http://www.nursingqualtiy.org/About-NDNQI

Sewell, J.(2019). *Informatics and Nursing: Opportunities and Challenges*. Philadelphia: Wolters Kluwer.

Sheroff, J. (2012). *Improving outcomes with CDS support: An implementer's guide* (2nd ed.). Chicago, IL: HIMSS.

Smith, K., Welker, R., & Zeko, K. (2019). 5 Evolving Compliance Risks That Should Be On Your Radar. *Healthcare Financial Management*. May2019, p20-26.

Souza, N., Sebaldt, R., Mackay, J.,Provok, J.,et.al. (2011). Computerized Clinical Decision Support-Systems for Primary Preventative Care: *A Decision Maker, 6*(87).

Study suggests medical errors now third leading cause of death in the U.S. (2019, 10 1). Retrieved from John Hopkins Medicine, 2016: http://www.hopkinsmedicine.org/news/media/releases/study-suggests-medical-errors-now-third-leading-cause-of-death-in-the-us

Telemedicine defined. (2019, 10 1). Retrieved from American Telemedicine Association: http://www.americantelemed.org/i4a/pages/index.cfm?pageid=3333

Thede, L. & Sewell, J.(2010). *Informatics and nursing (3rd ed)*. Philadelphia, PA: Wolters Kluwer.

Whedon, J. M. (2016). Relevance of Quality Measurement to Integrative Healthcare in the United States. *The Journal of Alternative and Complementary Medicine Volume 22, Number 11*, 853-858.

5 Strategic Planning

5.1 LEARNING OBJECTIVES

1. Describe how leadership plays a part in strategic planning for an organization.
2. Define the steps of developing a strategic plan.
3. Identify the components of developing the mission, vision, values, and goals for a strategic plan.
4. Generalize ways in which to communicate a strategic plan.
5. Identify how strategic planning fits into health care compliance.

5.2 INTRODUCTION

Strategic planning is heavily rooted in healthcare compliance. Likewise, leadership in health care organizations has a significant impact on strategic planning processes. Strategic planning helps to move an organization toward common goals and objectives, but the definition of strategic planning differs among many healthcare organizations. This chapter will address the foundations of a strategic plan; developing the mission, vision, values, and goals of the plan; and communicating the strategic plan with key stakeholders. It will also explore healthcare compliance as it relates to strategic planning in healthcare organizations.

5.3 KEY TERMS

- Strategic Plan
- Mission
- Vision
- Values
- Operational Risk

- Regulatory Risk
- Financial Risk

5.4 LEADERSHIP AND STRATEGIC PLANNING

Leadership has a significant impact on the strategic planning of any workplace (Jabbar & Hussein, 2017). The foundation of leadership is often described as planning and vision. Developing a strategic plan helps leaders determine the direction and goals for the workplace to achieve its outcomes. The strategic plan also helps the leadership of any institution link the heart of the institution with its body or purpose (Jabbar & Hussein, 2017). Imagine a workplace whose employees did not believe in the leadership or product that the institution was developing or delivering. How successful do you believe this product would actually be? Would the leadership of this company ever truly be successful? Now, imagine a company with a leadership that involved the employees in the planning and vision of the product they were producing. How successful do you believe this product would be? Leaders often give direction for an institution, but employee buy in and involvement makes the institution overall more successful.

Its leadership is responsible for developing the strategic planning process and moving the institution toward the goals it wishes to accomplish. In strategic planning, leaders are often responsible for many different roles. These roles include the following:

- Preparing the environment for change
- Creating a leadership team that involves key players in the institution
- Developing a vision and mission that clarifies the strategy for the entire institution (Moesia, 2007)

Assuring these steps are followed will help the leadership of any institution establish a well-defined strategic plan and gain employee support and understanding.

5.5 FOUNDATION OF A STRATEGIC PLAN

When developing a strategic plan, an institution most often refers to its foundation. For example, if our company developed programs to educate healthcare professionals in underserved areas, our foundation would be the population we wanted to serve. How would we begin to lay the foundation for building a strategic plan, to serve our population? What stakeholders would we need to involve in order to identify all of our needs? What are our institutions' goals? How will we define success? All of these questions help us to identify our foundation for developing our institutions' strategic plan.

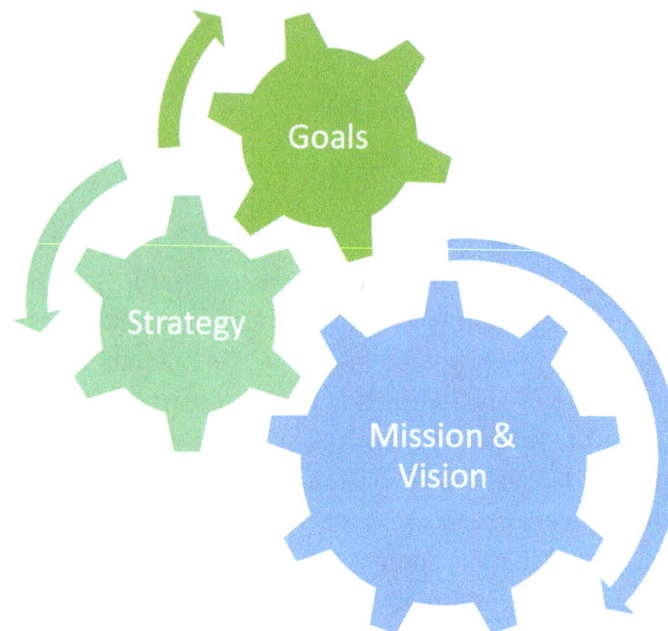

Figure 5.1: Foundation for Developing a Strategic Plan

Source: Original Work
Attribution: Sarah Brinson
License: CC BY-SA 4.0

Identifying stakeholders early in the strategic planning process helps the institution align its mission, vision, strategy and goals. For example, key stakeholders in our company who are developing programs to educate healthcare professionals in underserved areas would involve institutions of higher education, healthcare facilities and partners, community partners, technology partners, and publishing partners. Involving these stakeholders in our institutions' strategies and goals will help us better define our success.

An example of a goal and strategy for our imaginary company that will develop programs to educate healthcare professionals in underserved areas could look something like this:

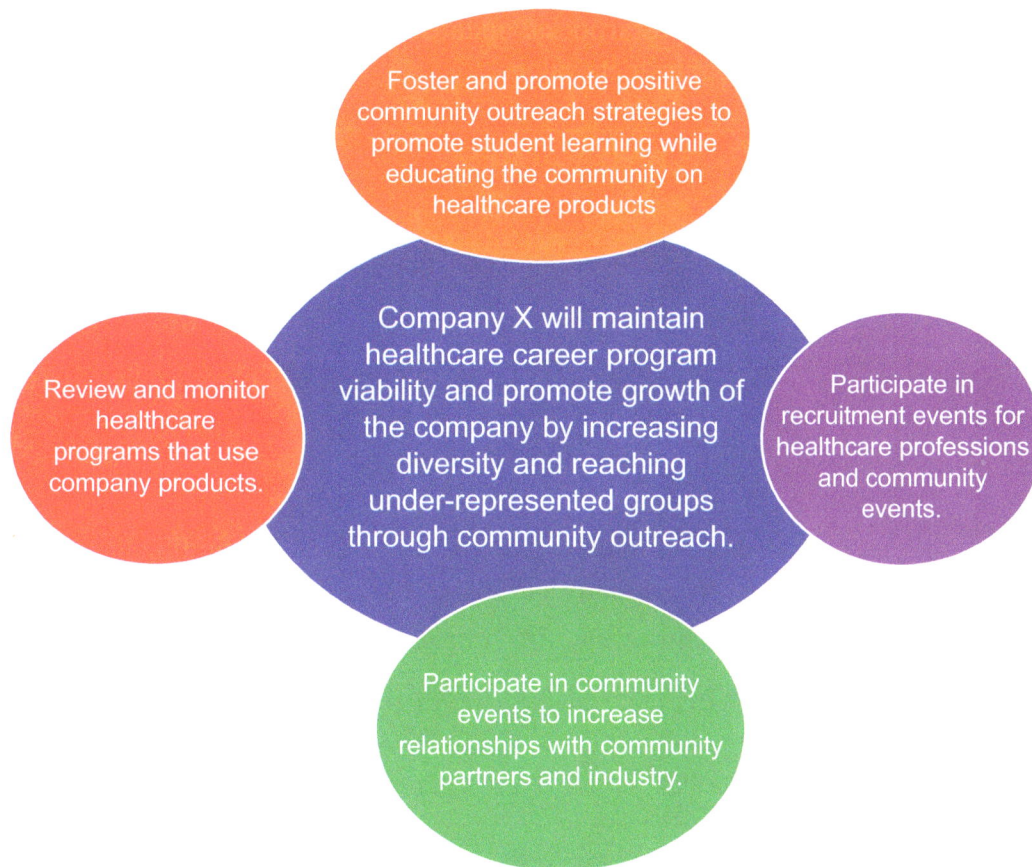

Figure 5.2: An Example of a Goal and Strategy for Company X

Here, the large middle circle represents the company's goal, while the outside circles represent the company's strategies and actions for reaching this goal.

5.6 MISSION, VISION, VALUES, AND GOALS

Once an institution's leadership has employee and stakeholder support, the strategic plan development process can begin. This process begins by developing the mission, vision, values and goals for the institution.

5.6.1 Mission and Values

An institution's mission often relates to its overarching purpose and is typically communicated with the entire institution, its stakeholders, and the public in written form. A mission statement answers the questions of who the institution is, what they do and value, and how they would like to move forward in the future. A mission statement communicates the institution's reason for being and how it plans to serve its key stakeholders. Some mission statements also include the institution's values or beliefs. For example, the mission statement from the international coffee company Starbucks, updated in 2019, includes four guiding principles that also communicate its values.

STARBUCKS MISSION AND VALUES

OUR MISSION

> *To inspire and nurture the human spirit – one person, one cup, and one neighborhood at a time.*

OUR VALUES

With our partners, our coffee, and our customers at our core, we live these values:

- Creating a culture of warmth and belonging, where everyone is welcome.

- Acting with courage, challenging the status quo, and finding new ways to grow our company and each other.

- Being present, connecting with transparency, dignity, and respect.

- Delivering our very best in all we do, holding ourselves accountable for results.

(Starbucks website)

The mission of any institution needs to focus on several key areas, including the following:

- What service or commodity it wants to produce and work to improve?
- How to increase the wealth or quality of life of its stakeholders.
- How to provide opportunities for the productive employment of people.
- How the institution is creating high quality and meaningful work for its employees.
- How does the institution live up to the obligation of creating fair and equitable employee wages?
- How does the institution provide fair return on capital (O'Hallaron & O' Hallaron, 2000).

The mission statement should be clear and be used to show where the company wishes to go.

5.6.2 Vision

An institution's vision differs from its mission in that the vision identifies the future of the organization along with its aspirations. In many ways, you can say that the mission statement lays out the organization's purpose for being, and the vision statement then says, based on that purpose, this is what we want to become. A vision statement helps to create the desired image of your future institution. Do you want your company to be known for creating the next iPhone app? Is your vision to be known for the best group communication text app? Your vision statement will need to address your targeted environment and what you aspire to accomplish.

Your vision statement for the institution also needs to include the "big picture" of your company. For instance, your vision may be to provide an international group communication app, but your vision statement would not include specific strategies to get you to this goal. An example can be found in the Starbucks Coffee's corporate vision "to establish Starbucks as the premier purveyor of the finest coffee in the world while maintaining our uncompromising principles while we grow" (Starbucks website). Aiming to be the premier coffee provider means that Starbucks Coffee wants to provide coffee of the best quality (Gregory, 2019). According to Gregory, "the company achieves this component of its vision statement by continuing its multinational expansion as one of the largest coffeehouses and coffee companies in the world" (Gregory, 2019, p. 2).

5.6.3 Goals

The overall purpose of developing goals for your strategic plan is to establish an achievable action plan for carrying out your mission and vision. Many strategic plans have failed because they were too complex or ambitious (Pract, 2009). The individual goals may not address all of your institution's limitations, but they should put you on a path of improvement. These goals can be readdressed yearly if needed, as long as they relate back to your mission and vision.

Each goal should also have an action plan that describes what the company will do in order to reach each outcome. For example, Starbucks included in its vision several of its goals, including:

- Premier purveyance.
- Finest coffee in the world.
- Uncompromising principles.
- Growth.

Establishing goals can be put into practice as we begin to imagine a company that will develop programs to educate health care professionals. We could establish yearly goals or actions steps that will help us reach our company's mission. Some of this company's goals may be as follows:

- Company X will maintain healthcare career program viability and promote growth of the company while increasing diversity and reaching under-represented groups through community outreach.

- Company X will develop a high standard of excellence in teaching and learning by engaging faculty with education, training, and mentoring opportunities needed to meet the goals of the health care program.
- Company X will promote a student-centered focus that will foster success, learning and improved program completion rates for all healthcare program students.

5.7 COMMUNICATING THE STRATEGIC PLAN

Your company's strategic plan will serve no purpose without communication. As you can see from the many steps listed above, the development of a strategic plan involves much time and effort. You will waste your time and effort unless you communicate this plan with the stakeholders and people upon whom it will have an impact. Communication of your strategic plan should involve communicating upward, downward, across, and outward (Hambrick & Cannella, 1989). Upward communication involves persuading upper management of the internal mission and vision within the strategic plan. Communicating downward means enlisting the support of the employees within a company who will be carrying out the strategic plan. Communicating across and outward involves other areas within the company and stakeholders that will be affected by the strategic plan. For instance, in our company, we will need financial support from across our company to develop and implement our products, and communication outside our company for community and student involvement.

Many institutions and companies communicate their strategic plan in a one-page format called a "snapshot." This allows the strategic plan to be shared with all parties in a simple manner. An example from our healthcare company could be as follows:

20XX – 20XX

Company X Strategic Plan Snapshot

Mission Statement:

As an academic healthcare educator, the mission of Company X is to educate the next generation of healthcare professionals in a collaborative and inclusive inter-professional learning environment, while providing accessible and culturally competent healthcare and wellness education through evidence-based practice. Through innovative education, interdisciplinary care, and community-based practice initiatives, the company is committed to leading the way in improving community health and reducing health disparities.

Long Term College Goals 20XX - 20XX

1. Company X will establish and implement well-defined and published policies and procedures that utilize best practice in order to improve overall company operations.

2. Company X will develop a high standard of excellence in teaching and learning by engaging faculty with educational, training, and mentoring opportunities needed to meet the goals of the company.

3. Company X will promote a student-centered focus that will foster success, learning, and improved program completion rates of all healthcare program students while implementing exceptional advising strategies.

4. Company X will maintain healthcare career program viability and promote healthcare program growth while increasing diversity and reaching under-represented groups through community outreach.

5.8 STRATEGIC PLANNING IN HEALTH CARE

Strategic planning in healthcare is really no different than in the institutions we have discussed earlier in this chapter. Strategic planning in health care involves outlining the action steps to meet your organization's goals (Regis College, 2017). Many of today's health care models require a more patient-centered and value-based approach to health care (Regis College, 2017). Norris (2016) claims that "strategic planning helps a healthcare organization do a better job of focusing its resources and energy" (p. 1). This process can also help to identify strengths and weaknesses within a health care organization and, ultimately, to minimize those issues.

Perera & Peiro (2012) describe five indicators that, in combination, suggest that all healthcare organizations need a strategic plan. These indicators include the following:

1. Informed, demanding, and non-loyal patients and clients who have a right to choose their healthcare organization.

2. Increasingly skilled and professional competitors (facilities and physicians).

3. Due to economic crisis in certain areas, there are limited resources for production.

4. The overall focus has shifted from the product or service delivered to the patient's experience.

5. The increase in population has led to an increase in the size and complexity of the healthcare organization. (Perera & Peiro, 2012).

These changes in our health care environment are often the driving force for an organization's strategic plan. The strategic plan not only moves the organization forward but also helps the organization remain in the forefront of constant changes and challenges in the health care market. As Johnson asserts, "To be successful in the future, no matter how turbulent the path forward may be, organizations need to create a vision based on the best future assumptions they can identify" (Johnson, 2017, p. 1).

5.9 IMPLICATIONS FOR COMPLIANCE

Health care related laws and regulations remain a challenge for many healthcare organizations. Many hospitals and healthcare organizations have begun looking at healthcare compliance through a different lens. According to Cerrato, "Instead of looking at them as routine operational responsibilities, they are incorporating compliance into a carefully crafted strategic plan, one that not only reduces the risk of large penalties but may even provide revenue opportunities" (Cerrato, 2013, p. 1).

The healthcare organizations of today are faced with many different risks that can potentially keep them from reaching their goals as set forth in the organization's strategic plan. These include market changes, workforce changes, technology changes and aging population changes (see graph below).

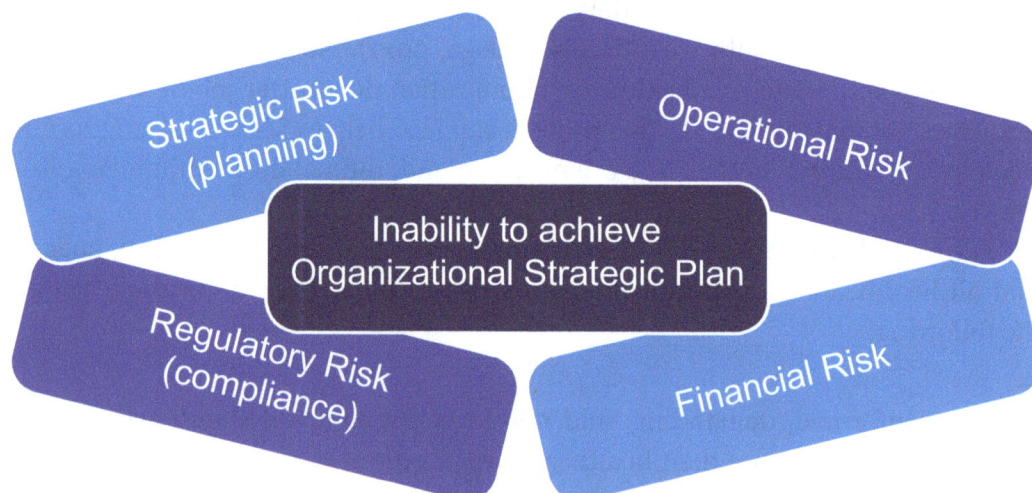

Figure 5.3: Potential Risks Preventing a Company from Achieving Strategic Plan Goals

Source: Original Work
Attribution: Sarah Brinson
License: CC BY-SA 4.0

Many healthcare organizations include compliance in the framework of their strategic plan. For instance, the strategic plan from Tuscola Behavioral Health Systems fiscal year 2017-2019 identified compliance as one of their "core strategies" for operation. Tuscola Behavioral Health Systems stated, "we will maintain a health care compliance system that will serve as a guideline for its good faith efforts toward compliance with state and federal regulations that apply to its services" (p. 9). Their strategic plan addressed compliance through the long-range initiative, goals, and objectives/challenges identified in the chart below.

#	Long- Range Initiative	Goals	Objective/Challenges
D. Compliance	Provide quality services within the guidelines established by regulatory and accrediting organizations.	• Achieve and maintain full compliance to standards/requirements from all governing, regulatory, and legal entities (including MDHHS, MSHN and CARF) • Ensure effective and secure use of the Electronic Health Record (EHR)	1. Achieve goals as defined by MDHHS, MSHN and other regulatory entities (QAPIP, BH-TEDS, MMPBIS, MSSV, KPIs, etc.). 2. Achieve effective administration of the annual Compliance Plan. 3. Ensure required and valid data elements are gathered via the EHR for reporting purposes. 4. Ensure effective and secure use of the EHR. 5. Complete the provider network monitoring to ensure compliance with contract and regulatory standards.

Table 5.1

Source: Tuscola Behavioral Health Systems
Attribution: Tuscola Behavioral Health Systems
License: © Tuscola Behavioral Health Systems. Used with Permission.

In many ways strategic planning and compliance seem to fit together in the health care environment. In this ever-changing and competitive environment, healthcare organizations are going to continue to find themselves amongst change and evolution. An organization's strategic plan and its compliance with established mission and values will help it venture through the waves of change and future growth.

5.10 SUMMARY

Strategic planning is often found at the core of many institutions and organizations. The leadership of an organization gives the direction and foundation for strategic planning from within the organization. Involving the employees of an organization in the strategic planning process helps to assure employee buy-in and helps to move the organization toward common goals and objectives that will make an impact on the company's outcomes. The strategic plan's mission, vision, values, and goals must be communicated throughout the company and with its stakeholders in order to be successful. Involving compliance with an institution's strategic plan will help the institution maintain healthcare compliance and will serve the institution's venture through the waves of future change and growth.

5.11 DISCUSSION QUESTIONS

1. How does an institution's leadership play a part in the development and implementation of a strategic plan?

2. Why is it important to involve stakeholders in the development process of your strategic plan?

3. Identify and define the important components of a strategic plan.

4. If you were in charge of developing a strategic plan for a company that created programs to educate healthcare professionals in underserved areas, with whom would you communicate the strategic plan and how would you communicate your plan?

5. Describe how an organization can include compliance in their strategic plan?

5.12 KEY TERM DEFINITIONS

1. Strategic Plan – a document that describes the direction of a company or institution.

2. Mission – a formal summary of the aims and values of a company, organization, or individual.

3. Vision – a description of what an organization would like to accomplish in the future.

4. Values – a statement that describes the top priorities of a company or organization and what its core beliefs are.

5. Operational Risk – the risk of a change in value caused by company losses that were not expected.

6. Regulatory Risk – the risk of a change in laws or regulations that may affect company operations.

7. Financial Risk – the risk that a company or institution may not be able to meet its financial obligation.

5.13 REFERENCES

Carriere, B., Muise, M., Cimmings, G., & Newburn-Cook, C., (2009). Healthcare succession planning: An integrative approach. *The Journal of Nursing Administration. 39*(12). pg. 548-555.

Cerrato, P., (2013). Compliance needs a shred strategic plan. *Healthcare Finance.* Retrieved from: https://www.healthcarefinancenews.com/news/compliance-needs-shrewd-strategic-plan

Gregory, L. (2019). Starbucks Coffee's Mission Statement & Vision Statement (An Analysis). *Panmore Institute.* http://panmore.com/starbucks-coffee-vision-statement-mission-statement

Hambrick, D. & Cannella, A. (1989). Strategy implementation as substance and selling. *The Academy of Management Executive. 3*(4). pg. 278-285

Jabbar, A. & Hussein, A. (2017). The role of leadership in strategic management. *International Journal of Research – Granthaalayah, 5*(5). pg. 99-106

Johnson, T. (2017). Strategic planning in the healthcare industry. *Balanced Scorecard Institute,* retrieved from: https://www.balancedscorecard.org/BSC-Basics/Blog/ArtMID/2701/ArticleID/1119/Strategic-Planning-in-the-Healthcare-Industry

Mosia, M.S. (2007). The importance of different leadership roles in the strategic management process. *S.A. Journal of HRM, 2*(1). p. 26-36

Norris, T. (2016). Why is strategic planning so important? *Healthcare Management Consultants.* Retrieved from: https://www.healthcaremgmt.com/why-is-strategic-planning-so-important/

O'Hallaron, R., & O' Hallaron, D., (2000). *The Mission Primer: Four Steps to an Effective Mission Statement.* Richmond, VA: Mission Incorporated

Perera, P., & Peiro, M., (2012). Strategic planning in healthcare organizations. *Cardololgia, 5*(8). 749-754.

Pract, J., (2009). Strategic planning: Why it makes a difference. *Journal of Oncology Practice. 5*(3). Pg. 139-143.

Regis College., (2017). Understanding Strategic Planning in Health Care Organizations. Retrieved from: https://online.regiscollege.edu/blog/understanding-strategic-planning-health-care-organizations/

Starbucks Coffee Company. https://www.starbucks.com/about-us/company-information

Tuscola Behavioral Health System. Strategic Plan, FY 17-18. Retrieved from: https://www.tbhsonline.com/images/pdf/Strategic-Plan-2018.pdf

6

Managing Healthcare Professionals & Strategic Management of Human Resources

6.1 LEARNING OBJECTIVES

1. Examine the management of different types of healthcare professionals in the workforce
2. Describe ways to manage conflict in the work setting
3. Identify ways to retain employees in the work setting
4. Define and describe the different components of human resource management in the workforce
5. Incorporate human resource strategies into the healthcare workforce

6.2 INTRODUCTION

Human resources management is a blanket term used to describe the development and management of employees in the workplace. The term human resources can be used to describe the department responsible for managing the resources of a company as it relates to the employees, or to describe the employees who work for an organization. Likewise, in healthcare compliance, human resource management includes the development and administration of programs that are designed to improve the productivity of an organization. This chapter will examine the management of different healthcare professionals in the workplace, conflict in the workplace, and employee retention. Incorporating human resource strategies into the healthcare workforce as it relates to healthcare compliance will also be explored.

6.3 KEY TERMS

- Management
- Human Resources
- Healthcare Workforce

- Conflict
- Employee Retention
- Employee Laws
- Employee Regulations

6.4 UNDERSTANDING THE MANAGEMENT OF HEALTHCARE PROFESSIONALS IN THE WORKFORCE

As healthcare systems throughout the U.S. and nation have expanded, increased attention is being placed on human resources management in the healthcare workforce. Human resources, as pertaining to healthcare, can be described as the management of the clinical and non-clinical staff responsible for providing particular health intervention (World Health Organization, 2000). The size, distribution, and composition within a county's healthcare workforce is often a concern (Kabene, Orchard, Howard, Soriana & Leduc, 2006). For example, the number of available healthcare workers in a region often defines the facility's abilities to provide health care. Many times in today's society, economic factors play a large part in the health care of a region or county.

The healthcare workforce is also an important factor to manage in human resources. Human resource personnel must consider the skill and training levels of employees entering the work force. They can do so by thinking about the hospital setting. For example, it would not be wise for an intensive care unit to hire all new graduate nursing staff who had no experience in taking care of patients in intensive care. Continued education and in-service training are often required to enhance classroom skills adequately for a real-world setting. A properly trained workforce is important for any healthcare setting.

In today's ever-changing economy, many organizations have implemented various health resource initiatives in an attempt to increase efficiency (Kabene, et. al, 2006). Outsourcing labor or hiring contract labor is often necessary to meet the needs of the healthcare facility and the region in which it serves. This strategy helps the healthcare facility ensure that it can meet the needs of its patients and work force. Other health care initiatives include attempts to increase equity and fairness as well as improving patient satisfaction with the care provided.

Human resource professionals face many different obstacles as they work to deliver high quality health care to their patrons and provide the needed support and training for their staff. Challenges such as budget, lack of support from stakeholders, values, employee attendance, high turnover rates, and employee morale all play a huge part in the everyday management of a healthcare facility. (Kabene, et. al, 2006). A solution to these challenges could be found through coordination of patient care and interdisciplinary teamwork (Kirby, 2002). According to Kabene, "Since all health care is ultimately delivered by people, effective human resources management will play a vital role in the success of health sector reform" (Kabene, et. al, 2006).

6.5 MANAGEMENT AND HUMAN RESOURCES

Employees are often considered the most valuable part of any healthcare organization in which a manager should invest. As Niles writes, "To develop a well-organized and competent workforce, the human resource management in health care organizations should provide constant improvement in such areas as job analysis and recruitment, legal and ethical management framework, health career promotion, distribution of employee benefits, motivation and support, and future trends in employees development" (Niles, 2013, p. 17). The partnership between the human resources department and management of an organization is often unique in the healthcare setting—including nursing—because many healthcare organizations are built on a multi-level managerial structure (Niles, 2013). For instance, the roles of clinical managers versus supervisors are sometimes confused. The clinical manager is responsible for the different aspects of a particular clinical setting, while a supervisor may be responsible for the entire unit. Human resources management often helps to bridge the gap between the different areas of healthcare.

One of the most important aspects of human resource management in healthcare is defining the ethical codes of conduct for the employees of a healthcare facility. Ethical codes of conduct must be developed for all healthcare facilities in order for employees to cope with moral dilemmas and conflict situations in the most efficient way. Many state and federal laws have been put in place to protect healthcare workers and patients. This legislature is often the foundation of the safety and welfare of healthcare facilities. The human resource's manager or department is responsible for laying the foundation for efficient standards that lead to a safe environment for all healthcare teams' members and patients.

Job analysis and design is also a foundational aspect of human resource management. Job design describes a set of duties and tasks that an employee will be required to complete in the workplace setting daily, while job analysis is the assessment of these skills performed by the employee. In order for the employee to be successful and continue to grow, job analysis from the human resources department or from the employee's manager is imperative. In turn, this process leads to efficient problem solving and decision-making skills by the employee.

6.6 MANAGING CONFLICT IN THE WORKPLACE

How conflict is handled in the workplace can make a difference in how employees feel about the organization moving forward. Human resource professionals are often given the task of handling or mediating employee issues. Along with managing these difficult situations, human resource professionals are also tasked with providing a solution to these issues that everyone can agree upon. You can probably imagine that finding a creative and strategic way of handling employee conflict on a daily basis cannot be easy. Forbes Human Resource Council (2018) recommends that allowing both parties to be heard, remaining transparent in the decision-making process, and finding a solution that makes both parties happy can make human resource management personnel better equipped to handle workplace conflict. The Forbes Human Resource Council (2018) recommends the following 14 strategies for mediating conflict resolution between employees:

1. Go in with an open mind
2. Be an advocate
3. Ask authentic questions
4. Remember you are the solution
5. Understand interpersonal effectiveness
6. Hear everyone out
7. Encourage open communication
8. Genuinely care
9. Help parties come up with their own solutions
10. Do not overcomplicate it
11. Reframe the situation
12. Stay focused
13. Follow up post-meeting
14. Coach for healthy conflict (Forbes, 2018).

There are no universal laws for managing workplace conflict. Every conflict has its own unique situation and outcome. Human resource professionals need to involve all parties in the conflict resolution process. Good working relationships often lay the foundation for successful companies, but even good working relationships are not always perfect. The overall goal of conflict resolution is to build a common ground to arrive at a solution for each conflict.

When conflict is allowed to go unresolved, it leaves employees and managers in a negative place. Not addressing conflict ultimately has a negative impact on productivity and teamwork in the workplace. In the end, it is up to the human resource management employees to determine the proper approach to addressing each conflict. Often everyone involved in the conflict believes their solution is the proper action. However, it is the human resource management team that must develop an in-depth understanding of the situation and what that led to the conflict in order to identify the possible outcomes that can help resolve the situation. Ultimately, the goal of the human resource management team should be to reduce or manage the conflict until a suitable resolution appears.

6.7 EMPLOYEE RETENTION

Finding employees who have the skills needed to work in healthcare is not the only challenge human resources management professionals face. Retention of employees is also a major concern of workplace managers. Many human resource professionals believe that it is easier to retain a qualified employee than to recruit, train, and orient a new employee to the same workplace. According to the SHRM's Employee Job Satisfaction and Engagement "The Doors of Opportunity are Open" research report, employees identify the following five factors as the leading aspects of job satisfaction:

1. Respectful treatment of all employees
2. Compensation/pay
3. Trust between senior employees and management
4. Job security
5. Opportunities to use job skills at work

Retention of healthcare employees is often difficult in the healthcare industry due to employee burnout. The healthcare industry is often considered a high-pressured atmosphere that comes with many unexpected events each day. Whether you are a nurse, doctor, physical therapist, or transporter in the hospital, your daily schedule many never be the same, and your work hours are often more than the normal 40-hour work week. Stories and data abound in regards to how clinical practitioners and staff at all levels are feeling frazzled and overwhelmed at hospitals, physician practices, clinics, and other healthcare organizations (White, 2019). According to White, "Between high patient loads with little time to provide personalized care, dealing with data entry in electronic health records systems and long, task filled shifts, many doctors and nurses are not only considering leaving their current jobs, they are thinking of abandoning their career choice entirely" (White, 2019, p. 2).

In many different job settings today, stress is abundant in the healthcare workplace. This stress will always lead ultimately to job turnover and dissatisfaction. White (2019) states that "in an industry where staff can make or break patients' outcomes and experience, it's key to boost your employee retention rates to keep the best and brightest from burning out or quitting" (p. 4). White (2019) recommends the following four factors in retaining employees in the health care workforce:

1. Recognizing achievements
2. Giving workers a purpose
3. Providing employees opportunities to relax
4. Creating a positive culture in your organization.

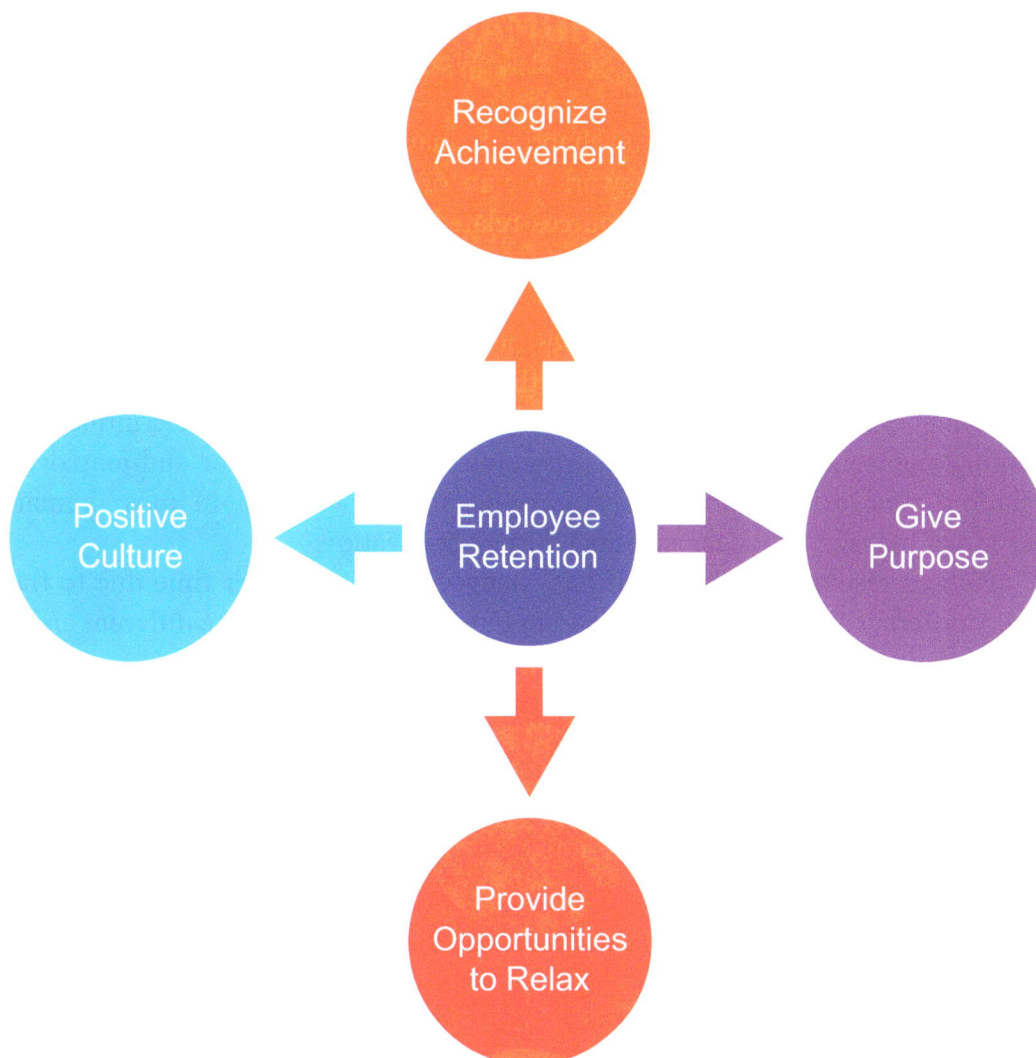

Figure 6.1: Four Factors for Retaining Employees in The Healthcare Workforce

Source: Original Work
Attribution: Sarah Brinson
License: CC BY-SA 4.0

Employee satisfaction and engagement in the workplace are often the key factors to employee retention. Imagine being in a job where your voice was heard and you had a feeling of belonging and purpose. Would you be more willing to stay in your environment and work harder? Would you stay in a job that did not value you as an employee and only considered you as a number? In human resource management, focusing on employee retention can lead to employee satisfaction, increased morale and quality of work. In the long run, employee retention and satisfaction pay off for the workplace: "The bottom line is that managing for employee retention, organizations will retain talented and motivated employees who truly want to be a part of the company and who are focused on contributing to the organization's overall success" (White, 2019, p. 1)

6.8 COMPONENTS OF HUMAN RESOURCE MANAGEMENT

As we discussed earlier in this chapter, human resource management is used to describe the employees who work for an organization and the department responsible for managing the resources related to an organization's employees. The term human resources was first coined in the 1960s when the value of employees in an organization began to take root. In today's corporate world, human resources management involves overseeing everything that relates to an organization's human capital—not just the employees, but the management and developments of all parties involved in the organization as well. Recruiting and staffing, compensation and benefits, training and learning, labor and employee relations, and organizational development can all be found in most human resources management departments for any organization.

Human resource management has changed drastically over time due to the many different areas that can be found in human resources. These different areas or career titles appear in the graph below.

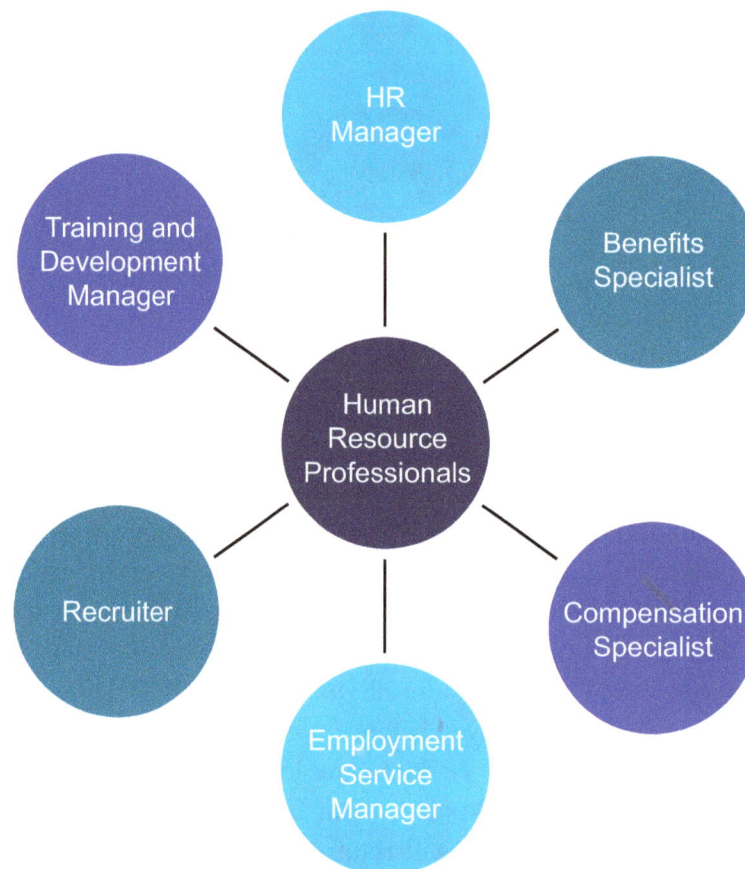

Figure 6.2: Human Resource Professionals

Source: Original Work
Attribution: Sarah Brinson
License: CC BY-SA 4.0

It is very common for human resource management professionals to possess specific expertise in one or more of these areas.

Developing or administering training programs that increase the effectiveness of an organization are also part of human resource management: "It includes the entire spectrum of creating, managing, and cultivating the employer – employee relations" (*What is Human Resource Management*, pg. 2). For most human resource management departments, the following list is included in their daily responsibilities:

- Managing job recruitment, selection, and promotion
- Developing and overseeing employee benefits and wellness
- Developing and enforcing personnel policies
- Prompting career development and enhancing job training
- Providing employee orientation
- Providing guidance for disciplinary actions
- Serving as the overseer of job site accidents or injuries and completing incident reports (*What is Human Resource Management*, pg. 2).

Along with overseeing each of the items above, the human resource management department must also be available to address employee concerns, help with the recruiting of new employees, oversee the employee separation process, and help to improve morale inside the organization.

Today's human resource management team is responsible for so much more than just managing people. In August of 2014, Forbes described the shifting changes and challenges in today's human resource management teams. The article discussed that human resource management teams must be able to communicate the vision and mission of the organization in order to have an impact on its organization and employees. Forbes (2014) suggested that the human resource management team of the future must focus on the following five critical areas:

1. *Define and align organizational purpose:* An organization's employees must be able to communicate the mission and vision of the organization. They must also understand how their efforts align with the organization's purpose.

2. *Recruit the best talent*: An organization must find an employee who has not only the skills needed to complete the job but also the personality and teamwork skills that will align with the current organization's team.

3. *Focus on employee strengths*: Organizations must understand what their employees do best and put them in positions where they can use their strengths.

4. ***Create organizational alignment***: An organization's achievements must align with its objectives.

5. ***Accurately measure the same things***: All departments within the organization must measure the same things in order to establish definite organizational results (Forbes, 2014).

6.9 ALIGNING HUMAN RESOURCE STRATEGIES WITH THE HEALTH CARE WORKFORCE

In order for health care management to work in a health care setting, human resource managers must align themselves with health care workers. Pastore & Clavelle (2017) claim that as health care systems change, the synergy in practice between human resource professionals and health care workers is an essential function of an organization's success. Let's consider Florence Nightingale, who wrote the Nightingale pledge for nurses. In 1854, while delivering care for British soldiers, Nightingale observed the overcrowded and unclean conditions of the military hospital. She used her observations to educate her fellow nurses in developing ways in which to improve the hospital environment for these soldiers, which in turn led to decreased infections and mortality rates. Nightingale used her care and compassion for these soldiers to better the outcomes of the hospital facility in which she served.

The relationship between human resource professionals and health care workers in the hospital setting is integral in allowing patient-centered care: "Organizational measurements on employee retention, management effectiveness, communication, and work-life balance can be traced to the early scientific analyses and experiments of Mayo and Nightingale" (Pastore & Clavelle, 2017, p.1). This partnership between health care workers and human resource departments lead to a strong and positive workforce.

6.10 IMPLICATIONS FOR COMPLIANCE

Human resource management and compliance is imperative for any organization to be successful. As discussed above, human resource management is often involved in the hiring and firing of employees, but the human resources of any organization also play a key part in the organization's compliance structure. Many different regulations and laws govern employment and employer-employee relations. A few of these procedures appear in the chart below.

Law or Regulation	Interpretation
Uniform Services Employment and Reemployment Rights Act (USERRA)	Gives certain rights to employees who are called to active duty.
Family and Medical Leave Act (FMLA)	Gives employees the right to 12 weeks of unpaid leave each year, under special circumstances, with the right to return to the same or an equivalent position upon returning from the leave.
Fair Labor Standards Act	Defines minimum wage and overtime pay for certain workers.

Table 6.1: Regulations and Laws Related to Human Resource

Source: Original Work
Attribution: Sarah Brinson
License: CC BY-SA 4.0

6.11 SUMMARY

Human resource management is a term that many different organizations use to describe the management of employees within an organization. Human resource management can include many different things within each organization, including the on-boarding and off-boarding of employees, employee benefits, employee training and education, the organization's compliance internally and externally, as well as conflict resolution. Today's human resource management team is responsible for so much more than just managing people. The relationship between human resource professionals and health care workers in the hospital setting is integral in allowing patient-centered care. Likewise, human resource management and compliance is imperative for any organization to be successful.

6.12 DISCUSSION QUESTIONS

1. Describe the management of different types of healthcare professionals in the workforce.
2. List three ways to manage conflict in the work setting.
3. Identify three ways to retain employees in the work setting.
4. Define and describe the different components of human resource management in the workforce.
5. What are some human resource strategies that can be incorporated into the workplace?

6.13 KEY TERM DEFINITIONS

1. Management- the process of running or controlling an organization or institution.

2. Human Resources- the department of an organization that handles the on boarding, off boarding, administration, and training of personnel.

3. Health Care Workforce- the workforce that is responsible for health care in hospitals, doctor's offices, and all other medical facilities.

4. Conflict- disagreement or argument.

5. Employee Retention- the ability of an organization or institution to retain its employees.

6. Employee Laws- defines employees' rights and obligations within the employer-employee relationship, wages, workplace safety, and discrimination.

7. Employee Regulations- regulations in statute law that establish minimum standards relating to the employment of persons, minimum working age, and minimum hourly wage.

6.14 REFERENCES

Efron, L. (2014). What Organizations Need Now from Human Resources. Forbes. Retrieved from: https://www.forbes.com/sites/louisefron/2014/08/18/what-organizations-need-now-from-human-resources/#18c16d33173f

Forbes Human Resources Council (2018). 14 ways HR professionals can solve workplace conflict efficiently. Received from: https://www.forbes.com/sites/forbeshumanreso urcescouncil/2018/04/10/14-ways-hr-professionals-can-solve-workplace-conflict-efficiently/#5a827a6c1250

Human Resource Edu. (2019) What is Human Resource? Retrieved from: https://www. humanresourcesedu.org/what-is-human-resources/

Kabene, S., Orchard, C. Howard, J.. Soriano, M., & Raymond, L. (2006). The importance of human resources management in health care: a global context. Human Resources for Health. 4(20), pg. 1-17

Kirby, ML. (2002). The health of Canadians – the federal role. In the Senate of Government of Canada Volume 6.

Niles, N. (2013). Basic Concepts of Human Resource Management. Burlington. MA. Jones & Bartlett Learning.

Pastore, G. & Clavelle, J. (2017). Healthcare HR and Nursing Leaders: Synergy in Practice. Healthcare Source. Retrieved from: http://education.healthcaresource.com/ healthcare-hr-nursing-leadership-synergy/

SHRM. (2017). 2017 Employee Job Satisfaction and Engagement: The Doors of Opportunity Are Open. Retrieved from: https://www.shrm.org/hr-today/trends-and-forecasting/research-and-surveys/pages/2017-job-satisfaction-and-engagement-doors-of-opportunity-are-open.aspx

White, J. (2019). Employee Retention in Health Care: 4 Keys to Keep Your Best and
    Brightest. Retrieved from: https://www.hrmorning.com/articles/employee-
    retention-healthcare/

World Health Organization: World Health Report 2000. Health Systems: Improving
    Performance. Geneva 2000. Retrieved from: http://www.who.int.proxy.lib.uwo.
    ca:2048/whr/2000/en/

7 Healthcare Technology

7.1 LEARNING OBJECTIVES

1. State the impact of improved medical technologies.
2. Explain the use of decision support tools for healthcare organizations.
3. Discuss the process of implementing an electronic health record in a healthcare organization.

7.2 INTRODUCTION

Rapid progress has been made to bring technology and the use of technology into the healthcare setting. Patient information can now be shared between providers, facilities, patients, and many organizations through the use of technology and electronic health records. Using technology not only improves the quality of patient care and efficiency but also can help in lowering the costs of healthcare. This chapter will discuss various topics as they relate to technology, including patient safety and quality while maintaining compliance within healthcare settings.

7.3 KEY TERMS

- HITECH Act
- EMR/Meaningful Use Data
- Data Security/Privacy of Information
- Interoperability & Interfaces
- Decision Making Support Tools
- Order Entry Systems
- Telehealth

Health Information Technology plays a vital role within the nation's quality strategy to achieve better care at lower costs along with healthy individuals and communities because advancements in technology enhance improving both patient safety and quality of care. In order to progress with better care and lowering costs—with technology—policies, regulations, and many programs are used to help transform healthcare. One policy we will discuss here is the 2009 Health Information Technology for Economic and Clinical Health Act (HITECH). The main goal of this act was to promote the adoption of health information technology and meaningfully use technology, the support for which it specified three phases of meaningful use (MU) for the nation's healthcare to achieve improved quality and patient outcomes. The Center of Medicaid and Medicare offered to give incentives to encourage providers and hospitals to adopt and use certified technology. In the U.S., the 2009 HITECH provided up to $26 billion in payments for hospitals and ambulatory clinics to purchase electronic health systems with clinical decision support (CDS) tools (American Recovery & Reinvestment Act, 2009). In addition to the federal mandate, organizations were required to meaningfully use electronic health records (EHR) technologies.

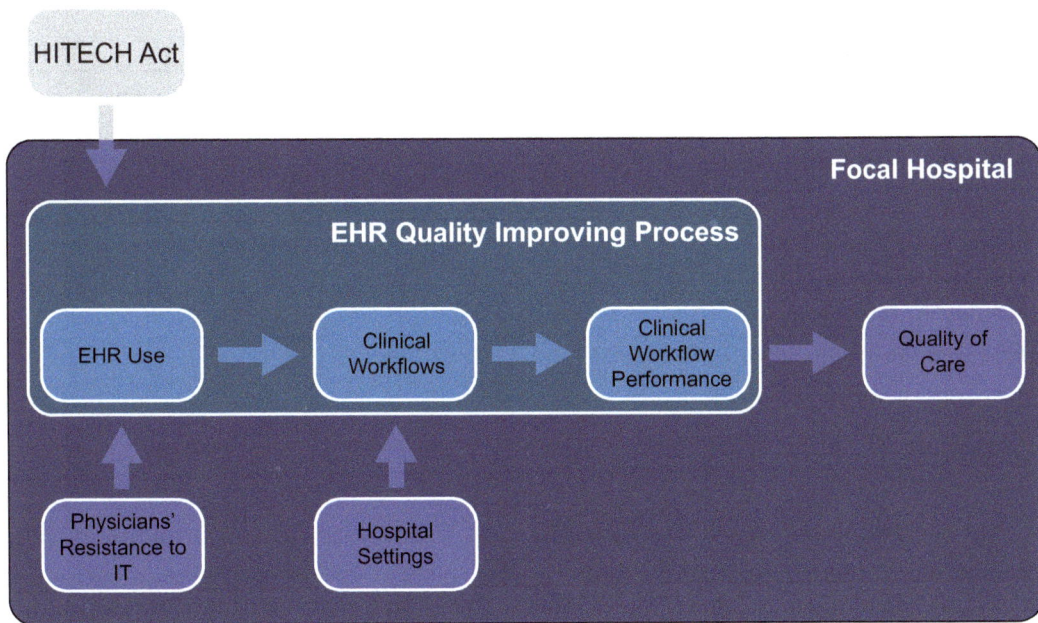

Figure 7.1: HITECH ACT

Source: Original Work based on Lin, Lin, & Chen, 2019
Attribution: Corey Parson
License: CC BY-SA 4.0

7.4 MEANINGFUL USE (MU)

In order to achieve the national strategy, the HITECH act (as noted above) specifies three phases of MU for the nation's healthcare to achieve improved quality and patient outcomes. Within each phase, advancements are made according to what is required from the capability of the technology. The table below delineates these phases, according to the Office of the National Coordinator for Health Information Technology (2018).

Stage 1	Stage 2	Stage 3
MU Criteria Focus on Basic Data Capture and Sharing	MU Criteria Focus on Advancing Clinical Processes	MU Criteria Focus on Improved Outcomes and Interoperability
Electronically capturing health information in a standardized format	More rigorous HIE	Improving quality, safety, and efficiency, leading to improved health outcomes
Using the information to track clinical conditions	Increased requirements for prescribing and incorporating lab results	Decision support for national high-priority conditions
Communicating the information for care coordination processes	Electronic transmission of patient care summaries across multiple settings	Patient access to self-management tools
Initiating the reporting of quality measures and public health information	More patient-controlled data	Access to comprehensive patient data through patient centered health information exchange
Using information to engage patients and families in their care		Improving population health

Table 7.1: Meaningful Use Information

Source: Original Work
Attribution: Laura Gosa
License: CC BY-SA 4.0

As we see from this chart, the first phase focuses more on the implementation of electronic health records and using the system to prescribe medications—electronically send prescriptions to pharmacies—and the ability to report quality data. The second phase focuses on patient engagement and the ability of the electronic health record to exchange data. The third phase focuses on value-based programs to achieve quality care and on supporting population health management. Throughout this MU program, hospitals and providers were financially incentivized with payments from the Centers for Medicaid and Medicare (CMS) if they implemented electronic health records and met the standards for MU. Additionally, there were disincentives in terms of payments for failing to reach MU. Starting in 2011, the incentive program continued over several years. As of April

2017, CMS had provided incentives for more than 523,000 eligible providers and to more than 4,900 hospitals with approximately $39 billion paid (CMS, 2018b).

Think About This Scenario

A seasoned provider has been using paper charting for his entire career in healthcare. Now, he has to learn the computer system for documentation and also the mandated requirements for MU to avoid penalties in payment from the CMS. He gets frustrated and so states that he "will stay on paper charting and the government cannot tell him what to do." His practice is in a large healthcare system. When reports are analyzed on the providers meeting the requirements, his name is on the list of "not meeting" requirements. How should the healthcare organization handle this? Should he be provided a scribe to help with his documentation? Should the organization offer to reduce his appointment schedule and have someone work with him one-on-one so he is more confident in using the EHR?

7.5 PATIENT SUPPORT TOOLS/DECISION SUPPORT TOOLS

One goal in particular to the meaningful use component is the implementation of tools that can guide providers in making appropriate decisions in patient care. These tools are called decision support tools. According to Campbell (2013), clinical decision support (CDS) is defined as a process to enhance health-related decisions and actions with pertinent, organized clinical knowledge and patient information to improve healthcare and healthcare delivery. These tools include reminders, alerts, clinical guidelines, diagnosis specific order sets, patient summaries, documentation templates, and referencing information (Greenes, 2014). The Institute of Medicine has recognized problems with the quality of healthcare in the U.S., and so advocates for the use of technology to improve quality patient care with such CDS tools (Sheroff, 2012). One goal in particular to the MU component is the implementation of tools that can continue to guide providers in making appropriate decisions in patient care. These tools are called decision support tools. According to Campbell (2013), clinical decision support (CDS) is defined as a process to enhance health-related decisions and actions with pertinent, organized clinical knowledge and patient information to improve healthcare and healthcare delivery. These tools include reminders, alerts, clinical guidelines, diagnosis specific order sets, patient summaries, documentation templates, and referencing information (Greenes, 2014). They help providers reach a proper diagnosis, ask the right questions, perform appropriate tests, prevent errors, reduce costs, and promote quality (McCool, 2013). CDS provides support at various stages of care, from the preventative phase all the way through the diagnosis phase, treatment phase, and monitoring and follow-up care phases (Berner, 2009). CDS intends to make data easier to understand, foster problem solving, process data, and assist providers in providing quality care. Many forces drive the implementation of CDS tools in a clinic, including the following: lack of a reference database within the application to facilitate providers in decision making, poor patient engagement with their healthcare, medical errors, lack of quality care, an increasing aging population with complex diagnoses, redundancy of tests, poor efficiency in workflows, high costs, and poor coordination of care (Greenes, 2014).

According to Greenes (2014), the efforts to stimulate the adoption of CDS depend highly on local needs and user preferences in many organizations, leading to difficulty in acquiring and little benefit in possessing CDS knowledge and experience. Rethinking the way our healthcare organization is structured needs our not only adopting CDS tools but also restructuring the information technology to support it—in order to achieve patient-centered care while focusing on wellness and to coordinate care processes (Greenes, 2014).

Also according to Greenes (2014), better informed decisions can lead to better patient outcomes. To facilitate this clinical decision making, information resources must be integrated into information systems. As clinicians use this built-in information, better decisions can be made regarding patient care. Additionally, clinicians will use information buttons ("I") as a point of care access to knowledge which will also automatically select and retrieve information from knowledgeable resources (Greenes, 2014). Integrated into the electronic medical record (EMR), the info button links can anticipate the information needs and also initiate the retrieval of information. Although it is available, it can be time consuming for providers to search for this information, which can be located within the areas of medication lists, problem lists, diagnosis areas, and orders areas. Further, to ensure MU adoption and their use of these buttons, they are included in every clinical guideline and quality measure (Cimino, Jing, & Del Fiol, 2012).

Other forms by which providers gain access to patient information within their organization's systems include the Epocrates monograph, which assists the provider and staff with more information on medications. UpToDate systems also compile information from experts who can assist with answering clinical questions. And apps on electronic devices assist providers with locating information as well.

Alerts are the most common form of CDS tools (Souza, Sebaldt, Mackay, Provok, et. al, 2011). Examples of end user tasks include the following: alerts, text messages and direct messages, notifications, and reminders within the system that alert the end user if an action is required. Medication alerts are extremely useful in offering a method to decrease adverse reactions. When medication orders are placed into the system, an alert can pop up for the provider if there is a contraindication or an incompatible medication. Alerts for patient quality measures are also extremely useful. For example, the patient may be due for a colonoscopy, so the system will alert the end user based upon the patient's age and the quality measure that the provider is using.

Such notifications and reminder tools are extremely beneficial to the healthcare organization. They could notify or remind the patient when it is time for a flu shot or to make an appointment with the provider; also, they can relay messages from the organization to the patient, including about outreach campaigns and health screenings. Notifications or reminders for the staff are considered part of the end user tasks, for example, with the user receiving a task that needs action, such as the notification that a patient's quality measure is due. However, if there is an impact to the provider's workflow or their time, CDS can lead to workarounds, ignoring warnings, and fatigue from their having to click through the alerts (Greenes, 2014). While such issues exist regarding alerts and reminders, many issues involve bypassing overrides. The system intends to assist with decision making; nevertheless, there continues exist many providers and staff who will ignore warnings within it.

According to Greenes (2014), CDS is a useful tool to apply medical knowledge to achieve great organizational performance. Greenes (2014) also discusses the CDS Five Rights, including that the right information must be presented to the right people, in the right formats, through the right channels and in the right points of workflow.

The organization must continue to optimize the deployment of CDS for maximum benefit and for the acceptance of its being utilized by the users (to avoid the problematic issues above). Greenes (2014) states that organizations should shift from viewing CDS as a built-in functionality within the system to viewing CDS as an added value that is incorporated into systems.

Figure 7.2: Clinical Decision Support Tools

Source: 123rf.com
Attribution: User "aurielaki"
License: aurielaki © 123rf.com. Used with permission.

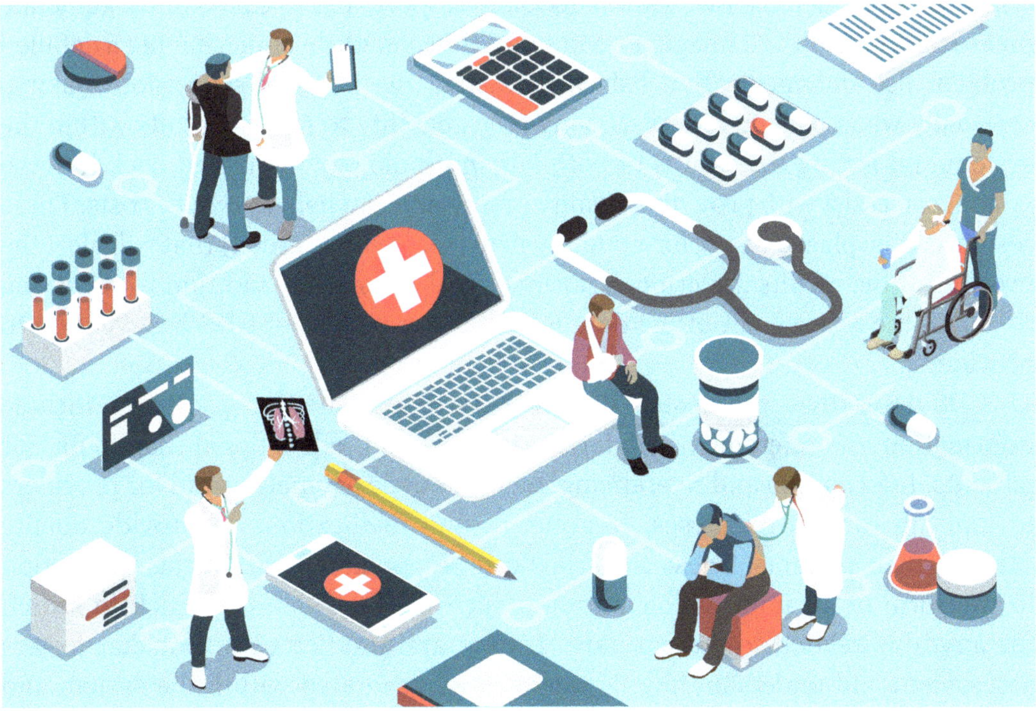

7.6 CLINICAL DECISION SUPPORT SYSTEMS

As noted above, the 2009 HITECH Act provided up to $26 billion in payments for hospitals and ambulatory clinics to purchase electronic health systems with CDS. In addition to the federal mandate, organizations must meaningfully use the electronic health records (EHR) technologies, including through CDS interventions.

CDS interventions can fall into one of four categories: data entry, data review, assessments, and triggers by end user tasks (Baker, 2013). Data entry includes smart forms and order sets that the system can use to help facilitate quality and improve efficiency for providers. Smart forms are an easy to use diagnostic and documentation tool that is especially useful to providers (Greenes, 2014). An example of smart forms within a system are flow sheets that allow the providers to look at results, vitals, and other pertinent data that can facilitate decision making over a period of time. These forms are easy to print and can also be used to graph the data that can be meaningful to the patient. Order sets are another example of data entry CDS intervention that can be particularly useful to providers. These ordering sets can be built by the providers or an informatics nurse who can generate a complete list of orders based upon a patient's diagnosis. Order sets are especially useful and also very efficient for the provider, saving them the large amount of time required to enter in many various orders.

Data review is a second form of CDS intervention and includes such items as reviewing accurate problem lists, medication monitoring, accurate allergy lists, critical results tracking, medication decision support, quality and clinical guideline measuring, and lab and imaging reviews. Within a medical clinic, having a detailed problem list and medication list can facilitate the provider's decision making, especially when placing orders. Having the capability to review results within the system and having the results of both lab and radiology interfaced back into the system can assist with providing quality of care and can help to reduce costs. These results can be placed in a color-coded system (red, yellow, green) that will alert the provider if the results are critical, normal, or abnormal. In addition to reviewing the data, the assessment of the data is a vital component of CDS intervention to providers.

CDS tools that can foster the assessment of data for providers include information or referencing material, letters, and educational handouts for patients. Information and referencing materials are extremely useful for providers to look up various diagnoses, treatments, and medications to provide quality care for their patients. These materials can be populated within the application in the form of an information button, which the providers can click to search for anything related to patient care. Letters are another CDS tool that fosters assessment and understanding. Letters can be generated within the system and faxed to the patient's primary care provider, specialists, or other providers that are a part of the patient's care team. This facilitates care coordination and allows the providers to communicate their findings based upon the patient's visit. Letters can also be sent to the patient's email using a patient portal system that can help engage patients in their care and keep them informed. Education handouts for patients are a component of meaningful use (MU) and are required by the provider to meet the MU measure. These handouts can be automatically populated by the computer based upon the patient's diagnoses or medications that are placed into the system by the provider. This function also allows patients to read and become more engaged in their care.

Lastly, such clinical professionals' tasks as alerts, text and direct messages, notifications and reminders are important CDS tools that would be extremely useful to patients, particularly in alerting their medical professionals that an action is required. Again, such alerts offer methods to decrease adverse reactions and foster patient quality measures. A huge component of these important alert systems is closed-loop ordering, which is where a provider can place an alarm on lab and imaging orders within the system. If the result does not return back to the system within the alarmed time frame, it will fall into a category of a "needs follow-up" so that the provider can investigate why the result did not come back. Often, it is secondary to patient non-compliance where the patient did not have the test or lab performed. Vaccine alerts are another useful CDS tool in which the provider can be triggered when it is time for the patient's vaccine. It is also useful if these vaccines are then interfaced with the vaccine registry system so that it is automatically updated and stays current.

As noted above, text and direct messaging are vital and beneficial alert CDS tools. They allow the provider to send a secure text message or a direct message via a secure email. Vital information can thereby be sent to facilitate the patient's care coordination, send consult notes to specialists, transfer care documentation between facilities, and foster communication between providers to enhance patient care.

Similarly, notifications and reminder tools for the patient or the end users can be beneficial to the clinic, as noted above, for such quality care measures as flu shot and appointment reminders. Also, the relay messages from the clinic to the patient regarding outreach campaigns and health screenings can be vital to ensuring increased patient care. Such notifications or reminders for the staff are considered part of the end user tasks. According to Carney, Morgan, Jones, McDaniel, Weaver, & Haggstrom (2014), such CDS alerts have significant impacts on cancer screening strategies which were improved using CDS alerts in community health centers. Patient engagement is considered a cornerstone for high-quality healthcare and can improve health outcomes for patients while reducing healthcare costs (Al-Tannir, AlGahtani, Abu-Shaheen, 2017).

Overall, CDS tools are extremely useful to improve safety, quality, care coordination, decrease medical errors, improve efficiency, and reduce costs (Sheroff, 2012). As Greenes writes (2014), there may be a significant cost savings when implementing CDS tools, especially if these tools fit well into clinic workflows and target gaps in healthcare.

7.7 TELEHEALTH

Telehealth refers to a range of health services that are delivered by telecommunications, such as through the telephone, videophone, and computer. The American Telemedicine Association defines telemedicine as "the use of medical information exchanged from one site to another via electronic communication to improve patients' health status" (ATA, 2010). The Mayo Clinic expects to serve over 200 million patients by 2020 using telehealth technologies (McGonigle & Mastrian, 2018). When information can be collected at home—through telehealth, for example—it can become more convenient for the patient and more productive for medical professionals. Telehealth can be used for patients with chronic conditions, at-risk patient populations, isolated patients, incarcerated patients, hospitalized patients, emergency response situations, home health patients, and employers and wellness programs.

Example

Think about a patient who has just been discharged from the hospital with new medication and a diagnosis of congestive heart failure. The home health nurse visits the patient twice per week. A home telemonitoring system was placed and tracks and transmits the patient's vital signs and weight. When abnormal data is detected in the system, the home health nurse can be alerted quickly and prompt a phone call to the patient. Also, the nurse can quickly contact the physician.

Telemedicine can prompt quick response times with early detections and timely interventions for patients. Research has shown that telemedicine can decrease patient hospitalizations and emergency room visits (Totten, 2016). However, telemedicine can also pose some compliance issues. A healthcare provider must be licensed in the state in which they are providing telehealth services and interacting with patients. Patients must also give informed consent to receive telehealth services and must understand the intrusiveness of in-home monitoring.

7.8 STANDARDIZED MEDICAL LANGUAGE

As the federal government pushes for healthcare organizations to adopt the use of electronic health records, there is a great need to have standardized languages between the systems. In order to facilitate accurate reporting, accurate data analysis, data extraction, and data sharing, many health systems work through interface messaging systems to map necessary data that may not equal each other. Having a standardized medical language within the systems allows for enhanced data sharing, which leads to evidence-based practice. In addition, when standardized languages occur between systems, the messages are easy to interpret and translate the data into meaningful pieces of information to other accepting systems. If standardization does not occur between systems, the messages would not be meaningful and the data could not be analyzed in a useful manner. Sharing data is crucial for the health of our patients. The sharing of data, therefore, must use standardized languages to facilitate the same meanings to downstream systems.

Think About This Scenario

A patient is seeing his primary health provider. The provider orders lab testing and also wants to refer the patient to a gastroenterology group for a colonoscopy, due to the patient's age, and this quality measure is populated on his electronic health record. The staff proceeds to draw blood for the lab work and the patient is told they would hear from the gastroenterology providers in regards to an appointment. Technology has now made it possible for the patient's lab results to be electronically sent back to the provider via the electronic health record, link up to the patient's chart, and also alert the provider for any abnormal results. The provider can also send the patient's progress note electronically to the gastroenterology group so they can follow up with the patient to schedule an appointment. Once the appointment is made, they can send a message to the provider.

Through the HITECH Act, this process was made possible. Such techniques streamline the chain of action so the provider can focus on the quality of patient care.

7.9 IMPLEMENTING AN ELECTRONIC HEALTH RECORD

The implementation of an EHR involves many benefits, including the following: improved efficiency, improved accuracy when performing tasks, immediate availability of patient records, and lower operational costs. Successfully implementing an EHR is more than just selecting a vendor and signing a contract. Project teams must be formed, organizational goals should be specific and acknowledged, and an implementation plan should address everything from hardware, workflow, training, and the required software for everyday tasks. Consequently, the process of selecting and implementing an EHR can be overwhelming if careful planning does not occur.

The selection and implementation process involves a great deal of time and costs, so the selection of an EHR should not be taken lightly. Many deciding factors should go into choosing the most appropriate one for the organization. The deployment of an EHR is not always just about the technology pieces that are involved. It also means finding an EHR that will assist the organization to reach their business objectives (McCarthy & Eastman, 2010).

Careful considerations should include the capability of the EHR to meet all of the MU requirements and appropriate safety standards as well as to offer quality measures, the best patient care standards, and solutions to the efficiency and the productivity of providers. When selecting an EHR, appropriate stakeholders in an organization should be involved. This step will save time and money when various vendors come to demonstrate their product to the organization. Of course, not every stakeholder has a lot of time to sit and listen to various demonstrations, so it is very important for analysts and information staff to research a few vendors before bringing them to demonstrate the EHR to only the stakeholders who would be involved with making the final decision from the selection.

In addition to managing the time involved during the selection process, managing time during the implementation process of the project is important as well. Developing a schedule is important when managing time during the implementation of the project. Scheduling requires some decision making on tasks to be done, the responsible party to perform the tasks, the time involved in the tasks, and any sequencing of the tasks that need to occur (Shirley, 2011). As already mentioned, stakeholders' schedules are an important part of managing time. They should be involved in the project, but their time should be respected, for instance, by not asking them to attend every meeting. Matching the project's tasks to the appropriate individual with the best skill set can be an important factor with timing. If this process does not occur, it may take an individual longer to complete tasks; it may also lead to inaccuracies. If a person with the appropriate skill set is not available, then extra costs to bring in consultants to help perform the task may be incurred (Shirley, 2011). Other time considerations include the sequencing of the tasks needing to be performed. This is important because it can cause a delay in the deployment of the project if certain tasks have to be completed before other tasks can begin. Careful planning, therefore, should occur, and each person should be held accountable for completing their tasks.

Taking the time to plan appropriately is important to the project's success and maintaining the project's timeline. Carefully analyzing the organization's workflow in the beginning phases of implementing an EHR can save time and money as the project continues to move forward. Every job in the organization must be analyzed to look for opportunities for improved efficiency—which may require some redesigning of workflows—so that the tools within the EHR can be used and maximized to its full potential. Managing costs are important when implementing the project as well.

The purchase of an EHR can be costly; however, the benefits can be worth the financial investment and can save money in the long run if managed correctly. Studies estimate the costs of purchasing and implementing an EHR range from $15,000 to $70,000 per provider (Fleming, Culler, McCorkle, Beckler, & Ballard, 2011). Each system may vary in the costs of the EHR. Besides the initial costs of purchasing the EHR and the time involved when selecting the EHR, other costs include hardware implementation, training, and maintenance costs. Some systems require organizations to pay per licensed user, some require a subscription with monthly charges, and others may charge a percentage per billed dollar amount.

It could seem favorable for an organization to go with the least expensive EHR software; however, this option may not be suitable for the practice and could end up costing more in the future. Consequently, developing a budget for these costs is important to determine if the project is on track. Estimating costs requires a lot of consideration of the project's resources, including people, materials, and the equipment needed to complete the project (Shirley, 2011).

In addition to the costs of the hardware and software, other costs to consider include paying for additional resources to come and offering training to staff. In a large organization, it may be suitable to pay appropriate consultants to offer training and support within the clinic on "go live" day. Also, data abstraction is a huge cost factor, especially for the clinics that are on an existing EHR and are changing to a different one. Entering in old patient data involves a lot of time. Costs can occur with data abstractions when decisions regarding who will preload the old existing data within the company arise, and may also ensue when hiring a data abstracting company to assist should extensive data abstraction be necessary. In addition to managing time and costs, project management also supervises quality.

According to Shirley (2011), project management, overall, is managing quality. The integration of health information is critical to provide quality care in today's fragmented health system. The EHR is a tool to facilitate quality, but it must be used correctly and to its full potential in order to do so. Otherwise, the stored information can become too cluttered and the providers will overlook it (Gill, 2004). The lack of real time information can result in delayed treatments, uninformed decisions, and medical errors. EHRs that have the capability to support disease registries and identify patients who need follow up care can report or audit to assist with managing quality through using work dashboards and facilitating a team approach to increase patient participation—all of which is important to managing patient care quality. However, whether it is the product's capability to manage quality or the quality of the project management process, quality itself is one of the most important tasks (Shirley, 2011).

Clearly, the selection and implementation of an EHR can be challenging. However, with good planning, strong physician leadership and involvement, and openness to change, the process can become less cumbersome (Smith, 2003). Managing time, costs, and quality are the most important factors for success with the overall project.

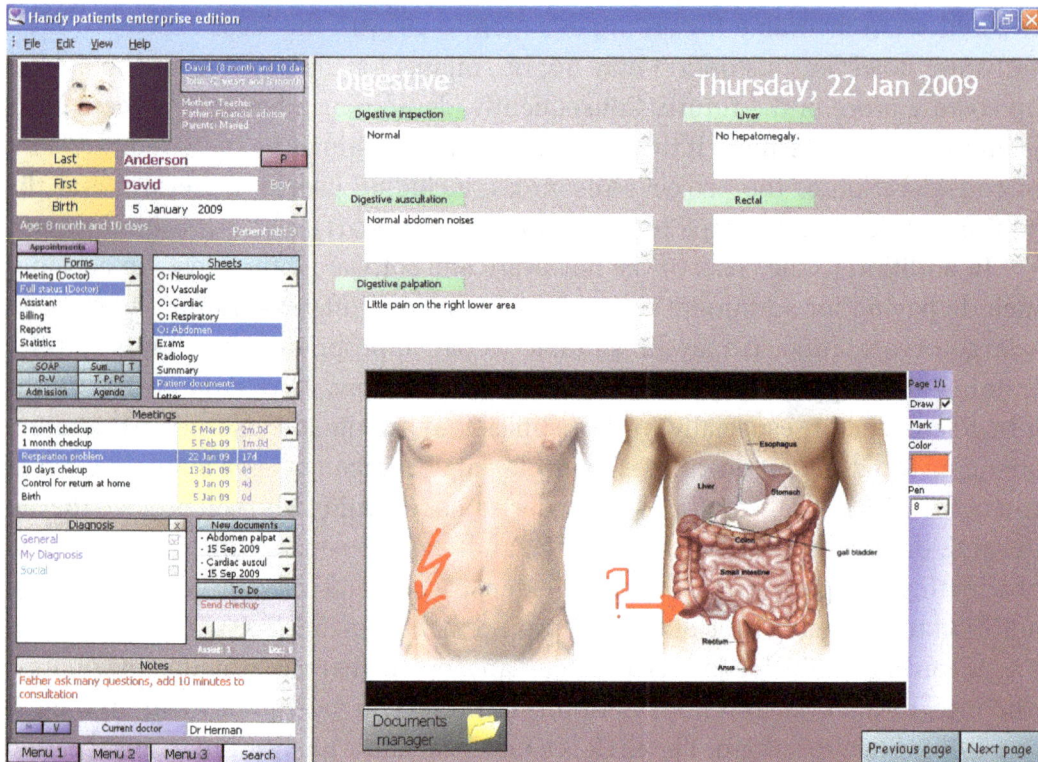

Figure 7.3: Electronic Health Record

Source: Wikimedia Commons
Attribution: User "DaCarpenther"
License: GNU General Public License

7.10 SECURITY

Security will continue to be an ongoing challenge in today's environment. As fast as new security measures can come out, hackers are quick to find ways to spread viruses and hack into the systems, so breaches in data still can be a problem. Many health systems thus utilize tools to monitor staff use and detect any breaches in data or confidentiality issues. Employees sending protected information via email must send it as an encrypted document. Each system used in the health system should have security measures requiring changing passwords within so many days. The computers and laptops have log off features, and many organizations have the policy to "control alt delete when you leave your seat." This phrase means to lock the screen or log off when walking away from the computer. Another concern that many healthcare organizations continue to have is nursing staff and providers' leaving the pull-down computers in the hallways open when they enter a patient's room so that anyone passing down the hall may view the charts. Managers must hold staff accountable if this incident occurs. For security, staff and providers are locked out of systems or roles are changed as needed when employees are terminated or transferred to other departments within the organization. Many organizations also have a data breach plan in the event that a data breach occurs. The rise in using EHRs has also caused security management to not keep up with the pace of healthcare data (Kwon & Johnson, 2018).

While the Health Insurance Portability and Accountability Act (HIPPA) was already in place, the HITECH Act also emphasizes the importance of data security, especially with exchanges in health information (Gold & McLaughlin, 2016).

Think About This Scenario

You are visiting your healthcare provider and the nurse is documenting your information into the computer system located inside the patient exam room. She then tells you she needs to go work up another patient and the doctor will be in shortly. She leaves the computer up with another patient's information displayed on the screen and you are able to view it. This is a huge HIPPA violation.

Here is another scenario: A patient visits the health care provider and the nurse clicks on the chart in the EHR but accidentally clicks on a different patient and does not realize it at the time. The doctor also sees the patient and begins to order some tests, labs, vaccines, and sends prescriptions electronically to the pharmacy via the system. Two days later, results come in for a patient that are abnormal, and the provider realizes that the patient was not seen and a different patient's chart was documented by accident. Years before electronic documentation, the paper chart could be removed easily and this mistake could easily be taken care of. Now, with the use of technology, the chart must be cleaned up. The pharmacy has to be notified and the patient has to be called to make them aware of the situation. The lab will need to be notified so the patient's results can to go into the correct chart. Not only will the chart within the healthcare organization need to be corrected but also the Georgia Registry of Immunization Transactions and Services (GRITS) will have to be notified and corrected because the vaccine registry was electronically sent via the EHR on the incorrect patient. If the patient had reminders or alerts scheduled on the patient portal system, it could also go out to the incorrect patient. This error can be a huge HIPPA violation in so many ways and also cause much stress when getting all the information cleared up within every system. When dealing with technology healthcare providers and staff must remain diligent to the chart they are documenting in.

The risks of violating a patient's privacy will always remain a concern when dealing with technology in healthcare. Electronic charting will heighten the risk of patients suffering the consequences of privacy breaches regardless of if such an action is intentional or unintentional (Agris, 2014). Protective health information should always be protected, and staff and providers must have extensive training on the use of EHRs and protecting patient information.

7.11 INTERFACES, HEALTH INFORMATION EXCHANGES, AND HEALTH INFORMATION ORGANIZATIONS

Interfaces enable a system to communicate and send messages to other systems, usually from a system to downstream systems. For example, a local health system has essentially two main systems; one is an EHR for ambulatory clinics, and the other is used for inpatient care within each hospital. Each system has a registration interface, a billing interface, and a document interface. Additional interfaces include laboratory and radiology orders and results. Each system has a patient portal interface where patients can log in and view their most recent clinical documentation. Also, dictation interfaces move the dictation to the transcription area and back into the patient's medical record. And there are interfaces with the Georgia Immunization Registry (GRITS) from each system to update vaccines.

7.12 SHARING INFORMATION

Increased healthcare costs, higher population ages, and struggles in today's economy are key reasons the healthcare industry must make changes in the way clinical information is shared (Jones & Groom, 2012). It is extremely important to communities that healthcare organizations come together and have access to data and shared information. Having a patient's medical history available anywhere and at any time is vital to support the health of our community. Indeed, the importance of a health information organization (HIO) is extremely vital to communities. This integrated data will help providers give a more holistic approach in patient care and will also allow the patient's big picture, health-wise, to be seen. Becoming integrated will require some effort in technology adoption, standardization, interoperability, privacy, and security in data exchanges to improve clinical and health outcomes (Jones & Groom, 2012).

Systems innovation in delivering information and reimbursement has increased stakeholders' needs to implement an HIO (Pina, Cohen, Larson, Marion, Sills, Solberg, & Zerzan, 2015). The continuous evolution of healthcare is why HIOs are important. Healthcare is moving to a value-based payment system, which is increasing the need to require health systems to integrate clinical data by pursuing alliances and partnerships (Kizer, 2015). Reimbursement is not the only important reason for the success of an organization to implement a HIO. Improvements in healthcare quality, efficiency, and patient engagement through a HIO are also important reasons for the success of an organization. Health care organizations will need the technology to help reduce paperwork and unnecessary treatments as well as decrease medical errors.

A robust infrastructure is required to support clinical integration (Strong, 2014). Many technical components are required to support data sharing. Interoperability is vital so that organizations can use data by communicating and sharing the terminology and definitions of relevant data (Jones & Groom, 2012). According to Jones & Groom (2012), there are three types of interoperability: technical, process, and semantic.

Technical interoperability refers to the hardware components needed to connect across a network and applications through simple exchanges, simple exchanges with a defined message, and complex exchanges. The technical pieces all work together to make sure the data is streamlined and shared between systems. Some of the components may consist of high speed, secure networks and the applications that have the capability to exchange data.

Process interoperability is necessary for communication between the systems to contain the appropriate data elements and to organize the data in a manner that will be meaningful to the end user. This process can include such components as an interface engine that sends data in a message format such as a health level 7 (HL7) message that will reduce data uncertainty and improve information transmission among all stakeholders. It can also include algorithms for patient matching and enterprise master patient indexes to ensure the data is correctly matched to the appropriate patient.

Lastly, semantic interoperability is vital for shared information. Jones & Groom (2012) define semantic interoperability as the capability of information shared to be arranged in an organized, sequential, and concise manner so that it is understood by the receiver—rather like the picture of the puzzle once the puzzle is put together. It can be sent in the form of a free text field; can be a form of classification, such as International Classification of Disease Codes (ICD 9 codes), Current Procedural Terminology codes (CPT codes), Healthcare Common Procedure Coding System (HCPCS), Systematized Nomenclature of Medicine (SNOMED codes), and National Drug Codes (NDC codes); and it can be sent as a blob of data elements that is meaningful to the end user or receiver.

Many key components are needed to implement the health information exchanges (HIEs) and health information organizations. Data sharing agreements, network access, interface engines and translations, record locator services, master patient indexes, data repository, standards, interoperability, data privacy, and data security are all necessary technical components for HIEs. Having all of these components is vital to the success of HIOs and to an organization. So why is there a great need to implement a HIO? To answer this question, one must look at the many benefits this system will provide. These benefits include higher quality and safe patient care, increased efficiency of providers, reduced costs, reduced duplicated testing, and reduced adverse drug events; they also promote better coordination of patient care and facilitate population health and disease management. Improvements in quality by sharing data can save between $70 and $80 billion annually (Centers for Information Technology Leadership, 2011).

Our nation's mission to use health information technology for the transformation of our healthcare system will be a challenging task. In order for the financial and clinical benefits to be successful, stakeholders will need to implement various small projects to progress the overall larger goal of HIO statewide as well as nationwide. As HIOs evolve, trust, collaboration, and communication are fundamental to a successful implementation (Penafiel, Camacho, Aistaran, Ronco, & Echegaray, 2014).

HIEs can provide various services specifically in Georgia. These services include the following: data lookup services and matching the patient to the data; secured data delivery and confirmation of the delivery; exchanging patient care summaries among organizations, including tests and the results; sending immunizations to the state registry; auditing data access and exchanging information; sending direct messages to providers regarding patient care; administrative services for claims and authorizations for treatments from insurance carriers; patient portals with clinical messaging; emergency access capabilities,; and exchanging data for disease management and community reporting. The goal is to have regional HIEs, then state HIEs, followed by a national HIE. What does this all mean? Basically, many health care organizations are partnering with regional health care organizations to connect and make a regional HIE so that relevant data is shared. For example, if you travel two hours south from where you live and get into a car wreck, the hospital there will have your relevant data, such as your allergies and medication lists, so as to treat you. As regions move forward with the development of HIEs, the state will have one state HIE where all healthcare systems can share relevant patient information for this same reason. It will be very similar to the GRITS platform which houses the state of Georgia's vaccines for patients. Lastly, the nation will progress into a national HIE. For example, if you travel to California and get in an accident and have no one with you to answer questions, the national HIE can be accessed to view relevant information to take care of you at that time. Huge, isn't it? There are still, however, many problems being worked out for regional levels before the HIE can progress to state and national levels. Having all of these services can improve the coordination of patient care and ultimately reduce the costs in healthcare. Clearly, HIEs are important for many reasons, but one main reason is due to the opioid crisis we are experiencing throughout our nation.

Years ago, providers were unable to view patient's information and would have the patient bring their pill bottles with them to their appointments so the providers could view what the patient was taking to document within their paper charts. Currently, systems are set up to allow the interoperability between EHRs and the Pharmacy Benefit Managers (pharmacy system) that will query and link up to anything the patient has purchased from the pharmacy. These systems allow providers to view medications accurately. However, there were some loopholes. The PBMs would only populate the data if the patient paid using their insurance card. So what do you think the patients who were seeking more medicine were doing? They were going to pick up prescriptions for narcotics and paying in cash so it would not be tracked. This practice led to huge workforce teams being placed on a project to get this problem corrected. So currently, any scheduled medications such as opioids will be placed into a database that can be viewed by any provider.

Pharmacies have to document this information into the system to include the patient name, date of birth, provider who prescribed the medication, when it was prescribed, and when it was picked up by the patient. This process allows providers to not prescribe a medication to a potential "doctor shopping" patient and to help in lowering the overuse of opioids. All of these solutions were made possible by technology and interoperability in healthcare.

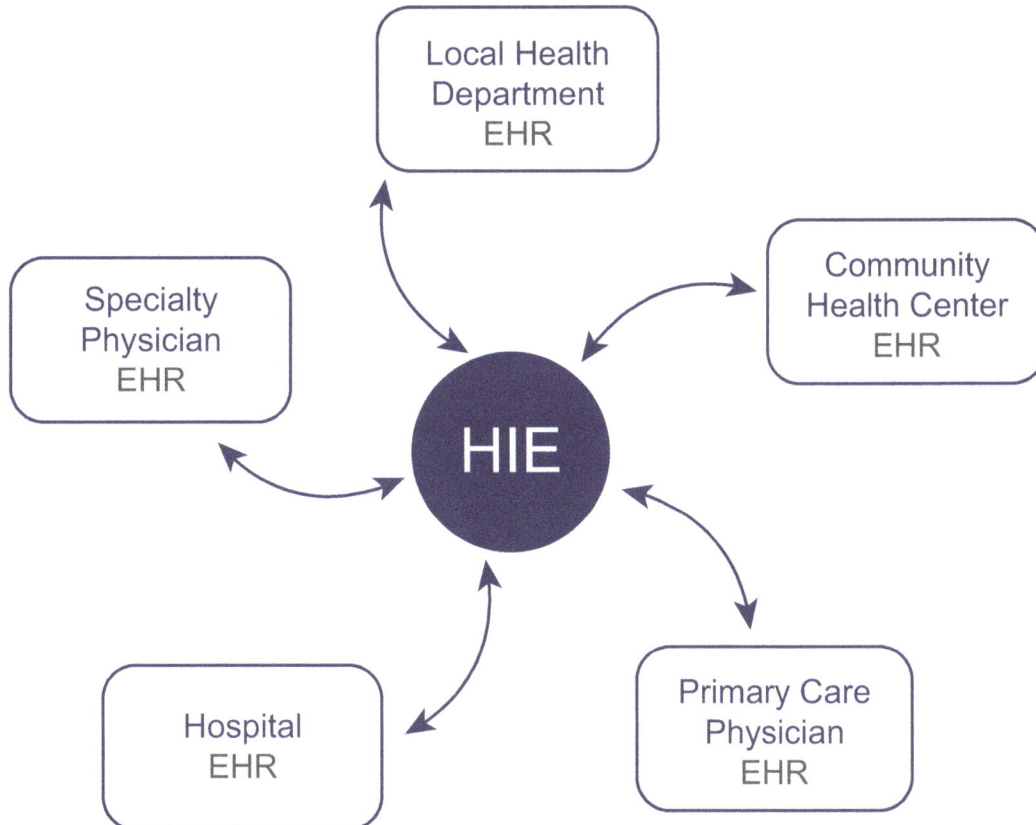

Figure 7.4: Health Information Exchange

Source: Original Work
Attribution: Corey Parson
License: CC BY-SA 4.0

7.13 IMPLICATIONS FOR COMPLIANCE AND SUMMARY

As the healthcare system is driven towards a value-based system, the need for better access to patient information and the ability to use and exchange patient information is vital to improve quality and lowering patient care costs (Thorpe, Gray, and Cartwright-Smith, 2016). Long gone are the days when paper charts were being utilized—to the point that facilities are being penalized for not having a certified EHR to document patient information. Schools must also teach using an EHR in all medical programs so students are better prepared to work and document within the EHR. However, schools of all medical disciplines must also teach paper charting. Because the EHR could go down for maintenance and upgrade, or simply have a glitch, staff will need to know how to document using both methods for such instances. Staff and providers must be trained to use healthcare technology and EHRs so that documentation is complete and thorough, and patient charts are easily trackable in noting who documented new information and when. Staff must also maintain such security measures as using only their passwords and not sharing passwords with anyone.

In addition to extensive training for using technology, providers must also know which areas of the EHR are mandatory fields to document information for billing purposes. Compliance departments in hospitals usually assist with training, alongside a nurse informaticist, to ensure that proper documentation is covered and staff know which fields of the EHR are used for billing and for quality management care purposes.

Staff and providers must be trained on viewing only the charts of patients for which staff and providers are responsible. Now more than ever, many staff members are fired from their positions and jobs due to curiosity. Years ago, staff only had access to the paper charts of patients they were taking care of on their floor or unit. Now, because of technology, staff are able to view any chart of any patient within the system. Consequently, more compliance audits are being performed throughout health systems.

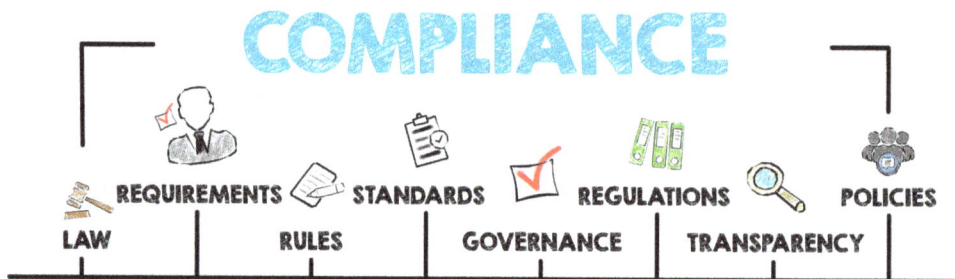

Figure 7.5: Healthcare Compliance

Source: 123rf.com
Attribution: User "tumsasedgars"
License: tumsasedgars © 123rf.com. Used with permission.

Think About This Scenario

A well-known famous person gets admitted to the hospital and comes through the emergency department for treatment. The patient then is admitted to the cardiac floor of the hospital. You are working in the hospital on another floor and hear some nurses talking and looking in the famous person's chart to see what happened. What should you do? Should you ignore the situation, report them, or confront the nurses? These situations occur now because it is so easy to view charts in the health system on any floor, unit, or department. It is imperative that staff only view the charts belonging to the patients for whom they are responsible.

Here is another common scenario: A nurse allows another nurse to use her password to document in a patient's chart in the EHR. The nurse who borrowed the password documents incorrect information, and now the patient has involved legal teams and support against the hospital. When the chart is audited, they are involving all parties that logged into the chart to document. The nurse states she did not document in the chart and she had given her password to another nurse who documented under her name. Should both nurses be held accountable? Why or why not?

Technology is vital in healthcare, but compliance must be involved to ensure that staff members are educated on its use while also protecting patient information. Privacy in the healthcare system is huge particularly because staff members have access to some of the most intimate information about a patient's health. Cybersecurity is another topic relevant to compliance. When health data is held or transmitted across networks, it must be secure due to medical records being targeted by cybercriminals. In these days, many cyber-attacks are happening in healthcare. In 2015, 113 million health care records were breached (Cashwell, 2018). This rise in cyberattacks and using technology requires healthcare facilities to focus on cybersecurity compliance, protection, and prevention (Cabrera, 2016).

7.14 DISCUSSION QUESTIONS

1. Why would it be important for users of an electronic medical record to protect their passwords? Should an employee be held accountable for situations in which a computer screen is left open for bystanders to view? Why or why not?

2. Should health care students be given an opportunity to document using an electronic medical record during their college experience before getting a job in the workforce? Why or why not?

3. Discuss healthcare exchanges and why they are important moving forward in healthcare.

4. List one example by finding an article on a cyber-attack in healthcare. Discuss the article and what the outcome was.

5. Define meaningful use and why it is used in healthcare.

6. Why is compliance and technology so important in healthcare today? Discuss education aspects, financial aspects, and quality of care aspects.

7.15 KEY TERM DEFINITIONS

1. HITECH Act- was created to motivate the implementation of electronic health records and support technology in the U.S.

2. EMR/Meaningful Use Data- the digital equivalent of paper records in health care.

3. Meaningful Use- using the electronic medical record in a meaningful way to provide quality of care to the patient.

4. Data Security/Privacy of Information- the process of protecting data from unauthorized access and without data corruption.

5. Interoperability & Interfaces- the ability of computer systems and software to exchange and make use of clinical information.

6. Decision Making Support Tools- a wide range of computer-based tools developed to support decision analysis and processes.

7. Order Entry Systems- replaces more traditional methods of placing medication orders including written, verbal, and faxed strategies via the computer versus paper methods.

8. Telehealth—enhancement to healthcare by using a variety of telecommunication technologies to deliver virtual, medical, health, and educational services to patients.

9. Clinical Decision Support Systems—health information technology system designed to provide medical staff and providers with clinical decision support when making clinical decisions.

7.16 REFERENCES

Agris, J. (2014). Extending the Minimum Necessary Standard to Uses and Disclosures for Treatment. *Journal of Law, Medicine & Ethics*, pp. 263-267.

Ahmad, F., Norman, C., O'Campo, P. (2012). What is needed to implement a Computer-Assisted Health Risk Assessment Tool? An Exploratory Concept Mapping Study. *BMC Med Inform, 12*(1), pg. 149.

American Recovery & Reinvestment Act of 2009. Retrieved from: http://www. govtractus/congress/billepd?bill=h111-1.

American Telemedicine Association (ATA). (2015). Letter to the Telehealth Workgroup.

Retrieved from: http://www.americantelemed.org/docs/default-source/policy/ata-comments-on-21st-century-telehealth-package.pdf.

Baker, D., Qaseen, A., Reynolds, P., Garder, L., & Schneider, E. (2013). Design & Use of Performance Measures to Decrease Low-Value Services & Achieve Cost-Conscious Care. *Annals of Internal Medicine, 158(1)*, pg. 55-59.

Berner, E. (2009). Clinical Decision Support Systems: State of the Art. Retrieved from: http://healthit.ahrq.gov/sites/default/files/docs/page/pdf.

Cabrera, E. (2016). Health Care: Cyberattacks and How to Fight Back. *Journal of Health Care Care Compliance.* September and October 2016.

Campbell, R. (2013). The Five Rights of Clinical Decision Support: CDS Tools Helpful for Meeting Meaningful Use. *Journal of AHIMA. 84*(10), pp. 42-47.

Carney, T., Morgan,G., Jones, J., McDaniel, A., Weaver, B., & Haggstrom, D. (2014). Using Computational Modeling to Assess the Impact of Clinical Decision Support within the Community Health Centers. *Journal of Biomedical Informatics, 51*(1), pg. 200-209.

Cashwell, Glyn (2018). Cyber-Vulnerabilities & Public Health Emergency Response. *Journal of Health Care Law & Policy, 21*(29), pp. 29-57.

Centers for Medicaid & Medicare Services. (2018b). Data and program reports. Retrieved from: https://www.cms.gov/Regulations-and-Guidance/Legislation/ EHRIncentivePrograms/DataAndReports.html

Center for Information Technology Leadership. (January 2011). The value of healthcare exchange & interoperability (HIEI). Retrieved from: www.hitdashboard.com/HIEI

Cimino, J., Jing, X., DelFiol, G. (2012). Meeting the electronic health record "Meaningful Use" criterion for the HL7 info button standard using openinfobutton and the librarian info button tailoring environment. *AMIA Annual Symposium Process*, pg. 112-120.

Fleming, N., Culler, S., McCorkle, R., Becker, E., & Ballard, D. (2011). The Financial & Nonfinancial Costs of Implementing Electronic Health Records. *Health Aff, 33* (3).

Gill, J. (2009). EMRs For Improving Quality of Care: Promise & Pitfalls. *Fam Med, 41*(7), pp. (513-515).

Greenes, R. (2014). *Clinical decision support: The road to broad adoption* (2nd ed.). Philadelphia, PA: Elsevier.

Gold, M. & McLaughlin, C. (2016). Assessing HITECH Implementation and Lessons: 5 Years Later. *The Milbank Quarterly, 94*(3), pp. 654-687.

HIMSS HIE Toolkit. (2015). Retrieved from: http://www.himss.org/ASP/topics

HIMSS Guide to Participating in a HIE. (2015). Retrieved from: http://www.himss.org/ ASP/topics_FocusDynamic.asp?faid=148.

Jones, S. & Groom, F. (2012). *Information and Communciation Technologies in Healthcare.* Boca Raton, FL: CRC Press.

Kizer, K. (2015). Clinical Integration: A Cornerstone for Population Health Management. *Journal of Healthcare Management, 60*(3), pp. 164-168.

Kwon, J. & Johnson, M. (2018). Meaningful Healthcare Security: Dose Meaningful-Use attestation Improve Information Security Performance?. *MIS Quarterly, 42*(4), pp. 1043-1067.

McCool, C. (2013). A Current Review of the Benefits, Barriers, and Considerations for Implementing Decision Support Systems. *Online Journal of NSG Informatics, 17*(2).

McCarthy, C. & Eastman, D. (2010). Change management strategies for an effective EHR implementation. Chicago, IL: HIMSS.

McGonigle, D. & Mastrian, K. (2018). *Nursing Informatics and the foundation of knowledge (4thed).* Burlington, MA: Jones & Bartlett Learning

Office of the National Coordinator for Health Information Technology (2018)Meaningful Use. Retrieved from: https://www.healthit.gov/topic/federal-incentive-programs/meaningful-use

Penafiel, C., Camacho, I., Aiestaran, A., Ronco, M., Echegaray, L. (2014). Disclosure of Health Information: A challenge of trust between the various sectors involved. *Revista Lativa De Comunicacion Social, 1*(69), pp. 35-151.

Pina, I., Cohen, P., Larson, D. Marion, L., Sills, M., Solberg, L., & Zerzan, J. (2015). A Framework for Describing Healthcare Delivery Organizations & Systems. *American Journal of Public Health, 105*(4), pp. 670-679.

Sheroff, J. (2012). *Improving outcomes with CDS support: An implementer's guide* (2nd ed.). Chicago, IL: HIMSS.

Shirley, D. (2011). Project management for healthcare. Boca Raton, FL: CRC Press.

Smith, P. (2003). Implementing an EMR System: One Clinic's Experience. *Fam Prac Management, 10*(5), pp. (37-42).

Souza, N., Sebaldt, R., Mackay, J., Provok, J., et. al. (2011). Computerized Clinical Decision Support-Systems for Primary Preventative Care: *A Decision Maker, 6*(87).

Strong, D. (2014). A Theory of Organization-HER Affordance Actualization. *Journal of the Association for Information Systems, 15*(2), pp. 53-85.

Totten, A. W. (2019, 10 1). *Telehealth: Mapping teh evidence for patient outcomes from systematic reviews. Technical Brief N. 26.* Retrieved from Agency for Healthcare Research and Quality: http://www.effectivehealthcare.ahrq.gov/reports/final.cfm

Thorpe, J., Gray, E., Cartwright-Smith, L. (2016). Show Us the Data: The Critical Role Health Information Plays in Health System Transformation. *Journal of Law, Medicine, & Ethics, 44*, pp. 592-597.

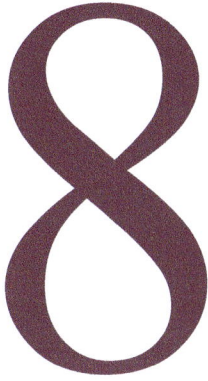

8 Special Topics and Emerging Issues in Healthcare Management

8.1 LEARNING OBJECTIVES

1. Identify emerging issues in healthcare.
2. Articulate the future of personalized health.
3. Analyze future challenges with health reform.
4. Describe potential future threats and challenges with the healthcare delivery system.

8.2 INTRODUCTION

The healthcare system is dynamic, constantly changing, and evolving. The continual emergence of technology has brought the rise of personalized health care. Changes in health policy and the political landscape continue to bring about changes in health reform. The ongoing strides toward improving healthcare cost, quality, and access brings evolution in the healthcare delivery system constantly. Healthcare providers and organizations should prepare for inevitable changes by forecasting potential challenges and issues that may arise in the future. This chapter will discuss special topics and emerging issues in healthcare management and their relevance to compliance in healthcare organizations.

8.3 KEY TERMS

- Population Health
- Person-centered Care
- Personalized Health care
- Health Reform
- Determinants of Health
- Personalized Medicine

8.4 EMERGING ISSUES IN HEALTH CARE

8.4.1 Population Health

Historically, healthcare has traditionally focused on treating health from an individual perspective. In recent years, there has been increasing emphasis on contributing factors that may impact community health, such as education, income, genetics, behaviors, and environmental exposures. The population health model acknowledges these different factors and how their intersection has an impact on health and focuses on improving health at a group level (Knickman & Elbel, 2019). The population health model refers to these factors as determinants of health. Determinants can arise from multiple sources, such as the following: (1) the social and economic environment, which includes income, education, employment, and social support; (2) the physical environment, which includes housing, availability of health foods, and air and water safety; (3) genetics; (4) medical care, which includes prevention, treatment, and disease management; and (5) health-related behaviors, which includes smoking, exercise, and diet (Knickman & Ebel, 2019).

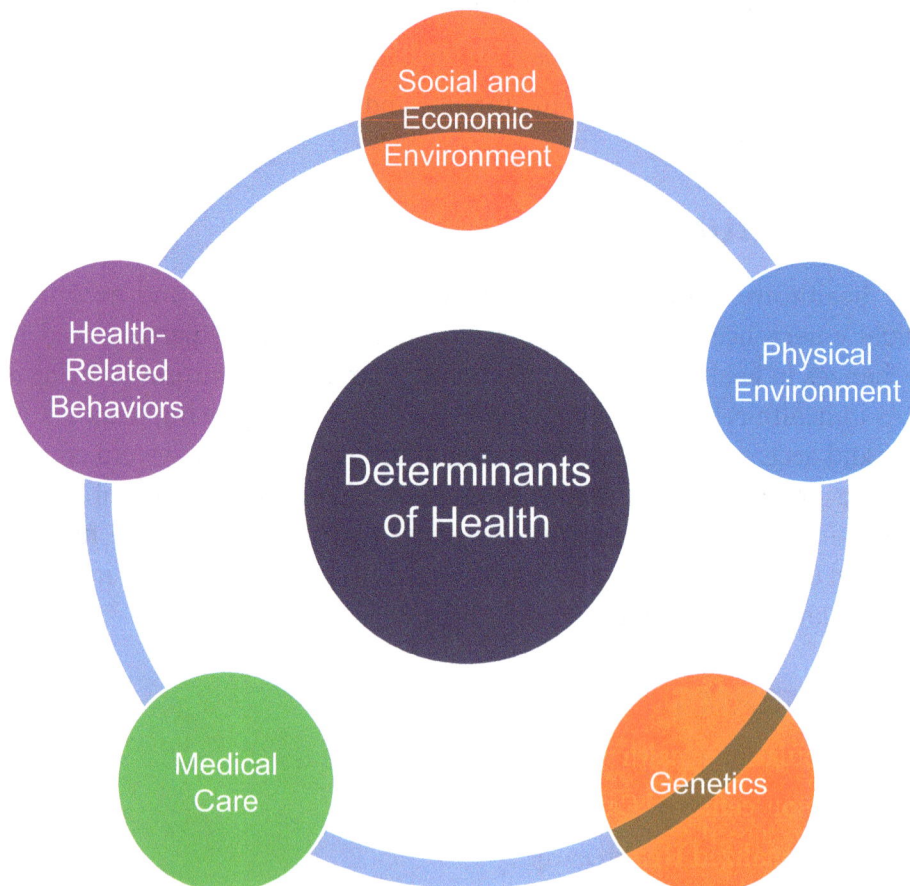

Figure 8.1: Determinants of Health

Source: Original Work
Attribution: Lesley Clack
License: CC BY-SA 4.0

Strategies for healthcare that strive to improve quality while also reducing the cost of medical care include appealing to payers, providers, and patients. Population health management refers to approaches that are developed in order to foster health and quality of care improvements for a population as a whole while managing costs (McAlearney, 2012). There are various types of population health strategies. Lifestyle management strategies aim to improve individual health habits and reduce health risks by using techniques to promote health behavior change from a health promotion or prevention standpoint. Demand management strategies utilize remote patient management tools in order to direct patients toward the most appropriate medical services. Disease management strategies attempt to provide medical care management services by focusing on a particular disease and providing services related to the needs of patients with that condition. Catastrophic care management strategies focus on providing the services needed by individuals who suffer from catastrophic illnesses or injuries. Disability management strategies attempt to bridge the gap between healthcare management and disability management in order to reduce lost worker productivity due to illness or injury. Integrated population health management strategies promote comprehensive health care for each member of a population by coordinating different health and care management strategies (McAlearney, 2012). Each of these population health strategies are designed based on specific goals and objectives that would best meet the needs of patients.

Real-Life Example: Disease Risk Management

Duke University Medical Center developed a telephone-based nurse care management program that was shown to improve medication adherence for African American patients with diabetes in rural areas. Nurses called patients each month for a year to discuss the patients' cardiovascular disease risk management. The conversations contained both standard and tailored components. The nurses' discussions focused on teaching the dangers of poor cardiovascular disease control, presenting risk factors clearly and credibly, and enforcing the saliency of the hazard. At each call, topics for discussion were chosen based on an assessment of the patient's knowledge and stage of behavior change. Nurses then contacted providers at three, six, and nine months to provide patient updates and to facilitate medication management. All nurses received training in community health, cultural sensitivity, and motivational interviewing. The intervention took place in community-based primary care clinics affiliated with an academic medical center.

The intervention has since been adopted statewide by the North Carolina Medicaid Agency and expanded to include additional conditions.

8.5 PERSON-CENTERED CARE

According to the Institute of Medicine (2001), the healthcare delivery system should revolve around the patient, respect patient preferences, and put the patient in control of their care (Joshi et. al, 2014). Person-centered care has become a major focus in healthcare delivery; thus, it is important to think about what types of services patients would like to see in the future. Table 1 provides results of a consumer survey conducted in 2018 by the PwC Health Research Institute.

78% of consumers stated that they are interested in having a "menu" of care options offered by multiple providers, which would allow them to choose care from local providers or virtual care from specialists across the country.
78% of consumers who had a hospital stay in the last 2 years reported that they believe at least a few of their recent in-person interactions with providers could have occurred virtually.
54% of consumers stated that they would choose to receive hospital care at home if it cost less than the traditional option.
54% of consumers stated that they would be likely to try an FDA-approved app or online tool for treatment of a medical condition.
47% of consumers would be comfortable receiving health services from a technology company such as Google or Microsoft.

Table 8.1: Current Consumer Health Care Interests (PwC, 2019)

Source: Original Work
Attribution: Lesley Clack
License: CC BY-SA 4.0

8.6 FUTURE OF PERSONALIZED HEALTH CARE

Personalized health care is a relatively new approach that is based on the scientific foundation of systems medicine that recognizes the dynamic relationship between genetic inheritance, environmental exposures, and systems biology. This type of health care uses the best predictive tools to identify each individual's health risks, the specific mechanism of their disease, and the best therapeutic approaches directed to their needs through health planning and coordinated care. Personalized health care can be used to enhance health, prevent disease, track its development, intervene early, and manage disease most effectively if it occurs (Snyderman, 2011).

Personalized health care and personalized medicine are terms often used interchangeably, but mean different things. Personalized healthcare is a broad term that includes any biologic information that helps predict risk for disease or how a patient will respond to treatments, while personalized medicine refers specifically to the use of genetics and genomics. An example of personalized healthcare is including specific biomarkers like lipoprotein that can help to better predict risk for heart disease or stroke in some individuals. An example of personalized medicine includes using specific tumor markers to guide therapy for breast cancer (Cleveland Clinic, 2012).

There are many benefits to using personalized health care. For one, personalized health care can improve the quality of care and decrease cost at the same time by helping us predict the right therapy with the fewest side effects for individual patients. Personalized health care can also help to engage patients in their care (Cleveland Clinic, 2012).

Real-Life Example: Personalized Health Care

Orlando Health uses large amounts of patient data to provide personalized communication to new mothers. Moms can choose a track to focus on—such as caring for a new baby or caring for family—and receive regular, personalized emails to address questions they may have. Instead of aimlessly searching the internet for help, new moms can get their individual questions answered right in their inbox.

8.7 CHALLENGES WITH HEALTH REFORM

Health reform is not a new concept; however, it will continue to take center stage for the coming years. Efforts towards creation of universal health coverage in the U.S. began in the early 1900s. Most of the other industrialized countries in the world have successful universal health care programs. Universal health coverage refers to a system in which health care is provided to all residents of that country or region. This is typically referred to as national health insurance (NHI), which is a health care financing system run by the government (Goldsteen & Goldsteen, 2013). The first NHI program appeared in the world in the 1880s, and most of the european industrialized countries had some kind of NHI system by the 1920s. The first campaign for a NHI program in the U.S. began in the early 1900s and was pushed by the American Association for Labor Legislation (AALL). President Teddy Roosevelt also proposed social insurance as part of his platform in 1912 (Goldsteen & Goldsteen, 2013). Over the years, many attempts at health reform were unsuccessful (table 2). Arguably, the most successful attempt at health reform in the U.S. was the Patient Protection and Affordable Care Act (PPACA) of 2010. However, as discussed in chapter 6, there have already been changes to the PPACA under the Trump administration, and we will likely continue to see changes. Health reform will continue to be a heavily debated topic in the coming years.

Year	Attempt at Health Reform
1912	Teddy Roosevelt and the progressive party endorsed social insurance as part of their platform, which included health insurance.
1915	The American Association for Labor Legislation (AALL) published a draft bill for compulsory health, which was initially supported by the American Medical Association (AMA), but the AMA reversed their position by 1920.
1930 – 1934	President Franklin D. Roosevelt appointed a committee to work on social policies to secure employment, retirement, and medical care but did not risk the passage of the Social Security Act to advance national health reform.
1935 – 1939	President Franklin D. Roosevelt pushed for national health insurance after the Social Security Act passed, but Congress did not support government expansions.
1944	President Franklin D. Roosevelt outlined the economic bill of rights in his State of the Union address, which included the right to adequate medical care and the opportunity to achieve and enjoy good health.
1945 – 1949	President Truman continued to pursue a national health program after the end of World War II, but the fear of socialism and power of southern democrats blocked all proposals.
1954	President Eisenhower proposed a federal reinsurance fund to enable private insurers to broaden the groups of people they cover.
1965	Medicare and Medicaid programs were signed into law.
1977	President Carter proposed Medicaid expansion for poor children under age 6, but the proposal failed to come to a vote in Congress.
1993	President Clinton's proposal, the Health Security Act, was introduced in both houses of Congress but gained little support.
1993	Other national health reform proposals were introduced in Congress but failed to receive sufficient support for passage. These proposals were the McDermott/Wellstone Single Payer Health Insurance Proposal and Cooper's Proposal for Managed Competition Without a Guarantee of Universal Coverage.
2006	Massachusetts passed and implemented legislation to provide health care coverage for nearly all state residents.
2006	Vermont passed comprehensive health care reform aiming for near-universal coverage.
2007	California failed in its attempt to pass a health reform plan with an individual mandate and shared responsibility for financing the costs.
2010	The Patient Protection and Affordable Care Act was passed.

Table 2: History of Health Reform in the U.S. (Kaiser, 2011)

8.8 WORKFORCE ISSUES

Currently, the U.S. is facing shortages in healthcare workers across the care delivery spectrum. According to the Association of American Medical Colleges (2019), the U.S. is facing a shortage of between 46,900 and 121,900 physicians by 2032. The American Hospital Association (2019) has reported that they support the Resident Physician Shortage Reduction Act, which is legislation that would add 15,000 residency positions funded by Medicare over five years in order to alleviate physician shortages that threaten patient access to care. Shortages are also prevalent in other healthcare occupations. An expected shortage of Registered Nurses (RNs) is expected to grow due to the increased aging of the population. The Bureau of Labor Statistics' (BLS) employment projections for 2016 – 2026 stated that the RN workforce is expected to grow from 2.9 million in 2016 to 3.4 million in 2026. The BLS report also projected that there would be an additional 203,700 new RNs needed each year through 2026. The American Association of Colleges of Nursing (AACN) is working with schools, policy makers, and nursing organizations in order to bring attention to this issue and is leveraging its resources to shape legislation, identify strategies, and form collaborations to address the shortage.

Another potential strategy for solving the physician workforce shortage is the use of mid-level practitioners, such as Nurse Practitioners (NPs) and Physician Assistants (PAs). An increased share of healthcare services are now provided by NPs and PAs. According to a New England Journal of Medicine study, the number of NPs and PAs nearly doubled between 2001 and 2016, and those trends are projected to continue through 2030 (Auerbach, Staiger, & Buerhaus, 2018).

Real-Life Example: State Approaches to Workforce Shortages

Iowa enacted a law in May 2019 that will provide opportunities for residency students to participate in rural rotations for exposure to such areas of the state. The University of Iowa will also conduct a physician workforce study on the state's workforce challenges related to recruitment and retention of primary care and specialty physicians. The study will examine current physician workforce data, identification of projected physician workforce shortages by region of the state, and analysis of the availability of residency positions, with an emphasis on the need for recruitment and retention of physicians in rural Iowa.

8.9 IMPLICATIONS FOR COMPLIANCE

Staying on top of emerging issues and trends is especially important in healthcare compliance. Practicing population health and person-centered care are both important to accreditation requirements. The ever-changing landscape of health reform brings about the need to comply with new laws and regulations. For example, personalized health care brings about an entirely different area of compliance, such as regulations on the use of genetic information. There are also future directions and trends in compliance. Organizations will integrate compliance programs from across the organization in order to increase efficiency. And compliance functions will use technology and data analytics more effectively for monitoring compliance issues (Deloitte, 2016).

8.10 SUMMARY

Many emerging trends and challenges in healthcare will potentially change the landscape of healthcare delivery in the future. Emerging issues such as population health and person-centered care change the ways in which providers interact with patients. New innovations such as personalized care have the potential to change the ways in which patients approach care. The ongoing debate over health reform in the U.S. brings with it a unique set of challenges, such as potential new laws and regulations that change how organizations deliver care. The challenges with adequate healthcare workforce impact all of these factors as well. These emerging trends and issues are all important to compliance; thus, healthcare providers and organizations should forecast for upcoming trends and changes.

8.11 DISCUSSION QUESTIONS

1. Discuss the difference between a population health approach to care delivery and a medical or individual approach to care delivery.

2. Your health insurance company informs you that they are now providing you with access to personalized live video doctor visits to assess symptoms, diagnose conditions, and write prescriptions. You will be able to get personalized care that addresses your unique medical history while still having the convenience of staying at home. Would you use this service instead of your regular physician? Why or why not?

3. There have been many attempts at universal health coverage in this country, and all have been unsuccessful. Do you feel that universal health coverage is possible in the U.S.? What would have to happen in order to be able to implement universal health coverage in the U.S.?

8.12 KEY TERM DEFINITIONS

1. Population Health- approaches that are developed in order to foster health and quality of care improvements for a population as a whole.

2. Person-centered care- care that revolves around the patient, respects patient preferences, and puts the patient in control of their care.

3. Personalized Health Care- use of any biological information to identify each individual's health risks, the specific mechanism of their disease, and the best therapeutic approaches directed to their needs through

health planning and coordinated care.

4. Health Reform- governmental policy that affects health care delivery.

5. Determinants of Health- contributing factors that may have an impact on health, such as education, income, genetics, behaviors, and environmental exposures.

6. Personalized Medicine- the use of genetics and genomics to predict risk for disease or how a patient will respond to treatments.

8.13 REFERENCES

American Hospital Association (AHA). AAMC Updates Physician Shortage Projections. Retrieved from https://www.aha.org/news/headline/2019-04-25-aamc-updates-physician-shortage-projections

American Association of Colleges of Nursing (AACN). (2016). Nursing Shortage. Retrieved from https://www.aacnnursing.org/News-Information/Fact-Sheets/Nursing-Shortage

Association of American Medical Colleges (AAMC). (2019). 2019 State Physician Workforce Data Report. Retrieved from https://store.aamc.org/downloadable/download/sample/sample_id/305/

Auerbach, D.I., Staiger, D.O., & Buerhaus, P.I. (2018). Growing Rates of Advanced Practice Clinicians- Implications for the Physician Workforce. NEJM Catalyst. Retrieved from https://catalyst.nejm.org/advanced-practice-clinicians-nps-and-pas/

Bureau of Labor Statistics. (2016). Employment Projections for 2016 – 2026. Retrieved from https://www.bls.gov/ooh/healthcare/registered-nurses.htm

Cleveland Clinic. (2012). What is Personalized Healthcare? Retrieved from https://health.clevelandclinic.org/what-is-personalized-healthcare/

Deloitte. (2016). New Horizons: Compliance 2020 and Beyond. Retrieved from https://www2.deloitte.com/content/dam/Deloitte/uk/Documents/risk/deloitte-uk-compliance-thought-leadership-16.pdf

Goldsteen, R.L. & Goldsteen, K. (2013). *Jonas' Introduction to the U.S. Health Care System, 7th edition*. New York, NY: Springer Publishing.

Joshi, M.S., Ransom, E.R., Nash, D.B., & Ransom, S.B. (Eds.) (2014). *The Healthcare Quality Book: Vision, Strategy, and Tools, 3rd edition*. Chicago, IL: Health Administration Press.

Kaiser Family Foundation (KFF). (2011). *History of Health Reform in the U.S.* Retrieved from https://www.kff.org/wp-content/uploads/2011/03/5-02-13-history-of-health-reform.pdf

Knickman, J.R. & Elbel, B. (2019). *Jonas & Kovner's Health Care Delivery in the United States, 12th edition*. New York, NY: Springer Publishing.

McAlearney, A.S. (2012). *Population Health Management: Strategies to Improve Outcomes*. Chicago, IL: Health Administration Press.

PwC. (2019). Top Health Industry Issues of 2019: The New Health Economy Comes of Age. Retrieved from https://www.pwc.com/us/en/industries/health-services/pdf/pwc-us-healthcare-top-health-industry-issues-2019.pdf

Snyderman, R. (2011). Personalized healthcare: From theory to practice. *Biotechnology Journal*, 7, 973-979.